Long-Awaited
CHILD

By Kellie Harriden

First Published: 2018 by Kellie Harriden
Author: Kellie Harriden
ABN: 55 133 661 590
Website: www.longawaitedchild.com
Email: info@longawaitedchild.com
Facebook: Long Awaited Child
Instagram: Long Awaited Child

Edited by: Bermingham Books
Designed by: Bermingham Books
Typesetting: Bermingham Books

ISBN: 978-0-646-99031-6

For Bane and Daya,

the babies I was meant to have.

CONTENTS

Difficult roads often lead to
beautiful destinations.

– Zig Ziglar

PROLOGUE

"So, when are you having a baby?"

The number of times we were asked this question was astounding. Trust me, I wanted a baby and every single time I was asked this question it got harder and more frustrating to answer.

Did I not seem happy? Did I have to have a baby to be happy?

I know no one meant any harm. This question seemed like a natural one to ask as I was in a long-term relationship, and 31 years old; as they say, "The clock is ticking."

INTRODUCTION

From first trying for a baby at 31 years old to finally holding my babies in my arms at age 39, I, along with my partner, Ian, went from many, many rock-bottom lows to some heart-bursting highs. Eight long and, at times, excruciating years might make some people want to throw in the towel, but we were determined to have a family—no matter how long we waited.

To this day, we still do not know why I was not able to fall pregnant naturally; however, during the time it took for our dream of having a child to come true, we knew we had to explore all possibilities. Nothing was a guarantee in the process, not until finally holding our

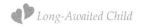

baby—well, babies (but we'll get to that later)—in our arms did we know for sure we would be a complete family.

All options outside of a natural pregnancy are expensive and emotional, and still provide no certainty for having a child. Over time, we explored all options after conceiving naturally was unsuccessful—in-vitro fertilisation, foster care, adoption, and surrogacy. It is said hindsight is a wonderful aspect, though it takes a situation to occur before that saying reaches fruition. Well, this book is my hindsight on our infertility struggles from first trying to have a baby to our baby joy eight years later.

I always thought meeting the right partner and then having a family together was how my life would naturally play out. I figured that motherhood was something I'd come to easily when I was a bit older and the time was right for me. It was not until I was in my early 30s and really ready to be a mum that I realised how much I truly wanted a family.

As our struggle became evident, I would witness family, friends, or even strangers having a beautiful moment with their baby or child and it would break my heart. I longed to have that same bond and unconditional love with my own baby.

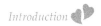

I was never really concerned with how I was going to have my baby; I did not necessarily need to be pregnant myself, just as long as I had a baby of my own to love. I remember back in my early 20s when a friend was pregnant with her first baby. One day we were catching up and she was devastated as her doctor had told her she would have to have a caesarean section instead of the natural birth she had planned. I kept my opinions to myself and consoled her, but to be honest I did not understand why she was so upset as to me it was the same end result — a baby of *her own* to love. I guess we all have our own ideas and dreams of when and how we want to have our own family and at times we all have to go down different paths to get to the same place at the end.

Chapter 1

OUR JOURNEY BEGINS

Our baby-making journey started in September 2004. It was an easy decision to start trying; Ian and I both knew we wanted a family. Earlier that year we had purchased our first home together in Tewantin. We loved our new home, had great jobs, and a good social life. Life together was good—but incomplete.

Ian and I met when we both worked in a resort on Hastings Street in Noosa Heads, on the Sunshine Coast in Queensland, Australia. I had not long returned to Australia after living in Ireland. Ian was the maintenance manager and I was the reservations manager. We worked together and occasionally socialised in the same groups for about six months before dating. The timing must have been right for both of us, as our relationship progressed quite quickly. Before we met, we had both travelled, lived, and worked overseas (well, in Ian's case, he bummed around the world surfing). I was almost 30 and Ian was 33 years old, and we both felt we had met the right partner to settle down with. Ian even bought me my first surfboard for my 30th birthday. According to him, this made him a keeper.

A few months after being together, we went on our first overseas holiday to Thailand, which was followed by many more exciting adventures. We enjoyed living on the Sunshine Coast and spent most of our free time at the beach. Not long after we had bought and settled into our new home, we started talking about having a baby. We decided there was no time like the present to start trying!

Was I the only naïve female in the world to think I would fall pregnant immediately upon trying? I had already planned a big announcement at our family Christmas gathering in a few months' time stating that Ian and I were expecting our first child. How was I to know any different? My sister had fallen pregnant with her three children very easily and, as far as I knew, my mum had as well. Within my circle of friends, whomever decided to try for a baby seemed to make an announcement of her pregnancy quite quickly, so why not me? Unfortunately, this was not the case for us, which is where our journey begins.

We started when I was in my very early 30s, an average time for many women. When you make the decision to have a child, many doctors will tell you, "Keep trying for 12 months and, if you haven't conceived after that, then talk to a doctor".

When we hadn't fallen pregnant within a year, we went to see our doctor. The first step was to have Ian's semen tested. When the results came back, the issue was not his semen. As Ian says, he was told he had the most excellent swimmers in all of the land. I am not sure those were the exact words the doctor used, but it's how Ian likes to remember it.

Before that test, the thought did not even cross my mind that I could be the one with the fertility problem. I was young, healthy, and fit, so I had no reason to think I would have a fertility problem. I just always thought we had our timing wrong and we were bound to conceive sometime soon.

I did have my moments after certain friends would

announce their pregnancy; it would hit me that it was not looking like it was going to be so easy for me. I was still very excited for my friends; as girls, we have our closest friends who we grow up with, dreaming of being pregnant at the same time so our children will grow up to be the best of friends, just like us. It really is ironic that I tried to avoid falling pregnant for so many years, yet when I was 100 percent ready to be pregnant, I was having issues.

Should I have spent my 20s in a relationship, with probably the wrong guy, just to have a baby at an earlier age when the chances of falling pregnant were higher? Having a family at a young age might have been the plan for some girls, and there is nothing at all wrong with that, but it just wasn't for me. I always felt I had all the time in the world. Instead, I spent my 20s travelling and living and working overseas. Whilst a lot of women I went to school with were having babies, I was living in some stunning locations, including Dublin, and holidaying on the Greek Islands. I had a blast and would not change those days for the world, and, to be honest, I never really felt ready to have a baby until I started to settle down with Ian. I would never have thought the girl having the time of her life in her 20s would have such a challenging journey to overcome in her 30s.

At the same time Ian was tested, the doctor also asked us a lot of questions to figure out if there were any small reasons why we had not fallen pregnant or changes we could make to increase our chances. Questions included our medical history, diet and exercise, alcohol consumption, the regularity of my periods, our previous sexual history, along with any birth control we had used.

There were not any issues there so the next step was for me to have blood tests to check my ovulation. These blood tests checked the follicle stimulation hormone (FSH)) blood levels; low levels may suggest there is less of a chance of a woman falling pregnant. My levels were slightly low so the doctor decided to put me on the medication Clomid (also known as Serophene or Clomiphene Citrate) as our first step. The medication would stimulate an increase in the number of hormones supporting the growth and release of mature eggs at ovulation. Taking Clomid can improve ovulation by 80 percent as well as increase the chance of falling pregnant by 50 percent in some women; however, no drug or treatment can offer a guarantee. I just had to take one tablet per day and endure the side effects, which, for me, were extreme headaches. But I continued, thinking if I was

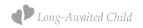

going to need assistance, I would just have to put up with some side effects, as this method was a lot easier and cheaper than other options.

After being on Clomid for around six months without a positive pregnancy test, we decided to go down the IVF path. You may be asking what IVF stands for and what it involves. In-vitro fertilisation, or IVF, is the process of fertilisation in which a woman's egg is combined with a man's sperm, usually in a laboratory dish. This will all take place at the hospital or clinic laboratory. To complete an IVF procedure, monitoring and stimulating the woman's ovulation with the use of hormonal medications is a necessary process. In order to extract the eggs from the woman's ovaries, the IVF specialist will conduct a minor surgery known as the egg retrieval. The eggs will be brought to a laboratory to be combined with the sperm to create embryos. The fertilised eggs undergo an embryo culture for two to six days before being transferred, or inseminated, into the uterus with the intention of establishing a successful pregnancy. This procedure normally takes place on the third to fifth day after fertilisation and the doctor advises the patient of the number of embryos to be implanted, which depends on certain factors like age. There are many reasons women seek pregnancy help through IVF, such as ovulation issues, male infertility, or damaged fallopian tubes.

Choosing an in-vitro fertilisation clinic can be a tough as there is such a vast choice. It is not just about choosing the right doctors and nurses at a clinic, but it is also putting your faith, trust and money into a situation to help you have the one precious little person you would treasure more than anything else in the world. To say it was one of our biggest decisions is an understatement.

One day, Ian and I happened to drive past a small clinic in Nambour in South East Queensland. I liked the quaintness and personal appearance the place portrayed as opposed to the bigger clinics, which gave me the impression that I would just be a number on the baby-making treadmill. As it turned out, we decided to go with this smaller clinic though the feeling that we might have made the first wrong decision on our quest bothered me for some time afterwards. Would I have had a successful pregnancy if we had chosen a larger clinic? To be honest, I did not know an awful lot about the processes of IVF at the time. I assumed all clinics would be following the same medical guidelines and the selection of a clinic really did not matter as the procedure would be the same,

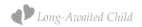

so long as we felt comfortable with our choice. After all, our contentment was the main point, right? The question of the right clinic, along with many other questions, has never been answered.

The next step after finding the right IVF clinic was to make an appointment to go through all the processes with the clinic experts to find what works best for us. Stepping into our Nambour IVF clinic for the first time was very surreal, but not in a good way. I honestly never in my life thought I would be there, but I was, and I was scared, nervous and underprepared. The staff were very friendly and made me feel relaxed in the unfamiliar environment.

As per the doctor's instructions, the clinic nurses provided me with the hormones I would need to inject into my stomach each morning and showed me how to do this myself. This was all planned to coincide with my menstrual cycle and the best time for me to ovulate. Leading up to the egg retrieval, I was advised to attend the clinic for regular blood testing to measure oestrogen levels and for scheduled ultrasound scans (camera probe inserted vaginally) to monitor how my ovaries were responding to the hormones. The doctors spoke about follicle stimulation hormone (FSH)) and luteinising hormone (LH), both unknown terms to me. They explained how the body produces the follicle stimulation hormone naturally to help the ovary prepare an egg for ovulation. In an IVF cycle, an artificial version of FSH is given to stimulate the ovary to produce multiple follicles (eggs) instead of just one. Luteinising hormone (LH) is another artificial hormone injection to control the timing of the follicle maturation and ovulation, which allows the doctors to perform the egg retrieval at exactly the right time.

At times, the doctors and clinic nurses seemed to speak in gibberish and acronyms that I was expected to understand, even though it was a very difficult situation and I was not an expert. Over the years, I told my clinic nurses to just tell me what to do and when to do it; I was not going to let any needles, blood tests, or the fact I felt every doctor on the Sunshine Coast was seeing my hoo-ha, bother me along the way.

I read some people find the injections horrific to do on their own and have to get their partner to do it. Ian left very early in the morning for work or was away for work so I really had no choice but to get on with it and do it myself. Trying to keep a full-time job and get out of work for doctor's appointments was the harder part for me; I had to try to explain why I needed to leave work early or needed to have an early lunch break for "personal" appointments. My career had mainly been in hotels and resorts and at the time I was in charge of group reservations at a busy resort on the Sunshine Coast. I was good at my job so, thankfully, I was never questioned on my need to leave work. No one at work was aware I was having infertility issues. I have never really liked the word infertility as it made me feel I was one of those women who were having problems falling pregnant. Surely I was not one of those women —I would be pregnant any day now, right?

After my injections of the hormones, I moved on to the egg retrieval process. This short surgical procedure was performed in the morning. After surgery I was monitored for a few hours, then Ian drove me home. At the same time as I was having my egg retrieval surgery, Ian was collecting his sperm. I am sure I do not need to explain what that involves; however, Ian was just relieved he could do it at home and not in a room at the clinic.

On the third day, after the egg and sperm were fertilised, the embryo was inserted into my uterus through a very thin tube (a catheter). It is important for the doctor to place the embryo(s) in the proper place. From there, I was told to just rest in order to not disrupt the uterus from too much activity. You hear stories of women lying flat with their legs in the air so the embryo does not fall out; though that is not true and cannot happen, a day's worth of bed rest is definitely suggested and I was advised to avoid any high impact activities or lifting until after the pregnancy test.

After the injections, the egg retrieval surgery and the embryo transfer, there was the dreaded two-week wait for the pregnancy test result. Anyone who has been through an IVF cycle will tell you this two-week wait is known for being the most excruciating part. The two weeks is to allow time for the embryo(s) to implant in your uterus. One major piece of advice I wish that I'd heeded was NOT going online looking for pregnancy symptoms! My patience levels were not the best during this time and this was one of my downfalls; if any pregnancy symptom was listed that my body did not have, I would convince myself I would have a negative test result. It was quite depressing and not worth the extra emotional turmoil. It's highly unlikely for women to feel or show any signs of being pregnant within the first two weeks.

When my two-week waiting period was over, I went to the doctor's office for my pregnancy test, which involved a blood test with the results the following day. Considering it was our first IVF attempt, I just assumed it would work the first time. Being under 35 years old, the success rates were quite good. As a woman heads towards 40, the success rate percentages head drastically south. Fortunately, with continued research, success rates have improved and continue to do so. There has been a lot of development since the first IVF baby was born in the United Kingdom in 1978.

The day I was to call the clinic for my test results, Ian was due home to make the call with me, but he was unfortunately held up at work in Brisbane. So, I had to put my big girl pants on and make the call to the clinic myself. I still remember sitting on the couch with the phone in my hand preparing to dial the number—I was shaking. I kept trying to convince myself it was going to be a positive result so all would be okay and I could celebrate with Ian when he got home. It wasn't! I do not think I have cried so loudly in my life. Seriously, I think all of the Sunshine Coast heard me. I could not understand how this did not work. I had done everything I had been told to. Why was this happening to me? Or in this case not happening for me? I was confused and alone.

Thankfully it was a Friday so I had the weekend to get myself together before going back to work. We had plans to visit my parents in Hervey Bay that weekend, as everyone was waiting to hear our result—it was not just us who thought we would be pregnant. Our families' anticipation and then surprise at our negative news was also very upsetting. Even though they were very supportive I felt like I could hear the disappointment in their voices. Telling them made me feel like a failure—like I was letting everyone down.

Chapter 2

DOING WHAT WAS BEST FOR ME

One thing I've learned about going through something important in life, such as this was for me, is the need for a tribe—especially for women. This tribe contains the people who have your back and will listen to your madness without any judgement whatsoever.

Sometimes the people we think would be "our tribe" are sometimes not, especially during trying times. I have heard of some women who discuss their fertility struggles with anyone—at the supermarket, at the school gate, pretty much anywhere anyone will

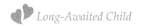

listen, as they may not have the support they need.

There is no right or wrong way to confront these issues or deal with every situation. For me, I just had to do what felt right for me and my own sanity. I felt every possible emotion during these times. One day angry, the next strong, to even feeling envious of any mum I saw with her baby. I started noticing babies and baby things more than I ever had in the past.

While I had plenty of support around me if I wanted it, but most of the time I was more of a loner and would listen to music, wallowing in my own self-pity. At other times, I would dance around the house trying to convince myself I had a handle on it all. Over the years, I pretty much had Sarah McLachlan's "Fallen" and Missy Higgins' "Everyone's Waiting" on repeat while I cried; for some reason, those two songs resonated with me. Even if listening to those songs made me feel even lonelier, it was what I did to manage my experience. To this day, I still love those two songs and they always take me back to that time in my life. I never want to forget the struggles Ian and I endured. I believe the obstacles I hurdled made me the person I am today—a strong woman who feels she can overcome any crappy situation thrown her way.

Ian was a great partner throughout. At times, he would purposely make me laugh when all I wanted to do was cry. He flirted with the nurses in the Nambour clinic to give me a laugh and they all loved him for it. One particular memory of an embryo transfer at the clinic still brings a smile to my face.

It was our second IVF cycle and we were in good spirits, believing it was going to work this time. We joked the first cycle was just a practice run. I was in my white hospital gown on the medical recliner chair as Ian stood in the room with me awaiting the nurses, who were in the laboratory next door ensuring the embryos were ready to be transferred. Whilst it was just the two of us in the room, Ian decided to play with the controls on the chair I was sitting on. He had me sitting up, laying down, legs in the air, back up and then legs up again—I could not stop laughing. The days before, during, and after an IVF cycle, especially with a negative pregnancy test, my thoughts were consumed with questioning everything in my daily life, so it was a nice relief to laugh out loud. Just as Ian was having the time of his life playing with the controls and seeing me laugh, the nurses entered the room. It was all very hysterical. But Ian knew how to make me relax and take my mind off things, for which I was very grateful.

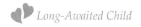

You see, I was very private with our baby-making journey. I was embarrassed that I couldn't fall pregnant naturally like my friends and colleagues. I started to feel like I was not only letting Ian and myself down, but also my family. My parents' grandchildren (my nieces and nephews) were all starting to grow up so fast and my parents loved the idea of a little baby being part of our family again. Feeling embarrassed was an outlandish emotion, which I know now, but I could not help the way I felt; not to mention, the hormones raging through my body created all sorts of irrational emotions that would pop up at any moment. Apart from some family and a few close friends, no one else knew what we were going through. I just never spoke about it and if someone asked when we were having kids, I just replied, "Not really sure" or "One day" or something like that to fob off the question, as though I did not really care if we had them at all.

When I eventually told my manager at work she confessed to feeling kind of relieved, as with all my "personal" medical appointments she thought I may have been terminally ill. Now, I do admit I may have had a couple of "extra" appointments just to get an early finish for the day. It was hard being at work when I was feeling emotionally drained and my mind was not on

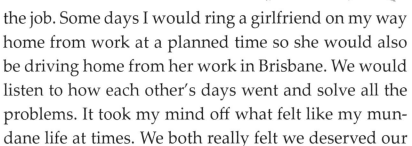

the job. Some days I would ring a girlfriend on my way home from work at a planned time so she would also be driving home from her work in Brisbane. We would listen to how each other's days went and solve all the problems. It took my mind off what felt like my mundane life at times. We both really felt we deserved our own drive home radio gig just like Hamish & Andy.

For some women, the doctor collects a good number of quality eggs during the egg retrieval process. This means the clinic can use the required number of eggs for that cycle and the remaining healthy eggs can either be frozen as eggs or fertilised and frozen as embryos. Then, if the client has a negative result with one cycle, she can try again by having just an embryo transfer without having to go through the hormone injections and egg retrieval surgery again. For me, it was not as easy. During each of my egg retrievals, only a small number of eggs were collected and, if there were spares, the embryos did not survive. This meant each IVF cycle had to be started from scratch—injections every morning, an increased hormone dosage to help increase the chance of more eggs being collected, and into surgery for the egg retrieval. Hence, my many, many appointments at the clinic. At times, I felt like I was having ultrasound scans and blood tests every

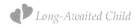

second day. It was not the most enjoyable time, but something I just had to do for the family I so wanted.

Our second and third attempts were the same procedure with the same negative result. When was it going to be a positive result for us? Life was starting to feel extremely unfair. On top of the financial costs, with each cycle I put on weight, a side effect from the hormones—not what I needed when already on an emotional rollercoaster.

At that point, I was willing to try anything to help reach a successful pregnancy test. Someone suggested acupuncture to me, as she had read an article about it helping IVF patients reduce stress, so I was prepared to give it a go. I booked in at a clinic near my home and had my first appointment after work one day. The clinic's interior was very white and had an overwhelming antiseptic feel; I expected a more serene room that would transport me to ancient China, but that was not the case. The acupuncturist who was going to stick thin needles in me greeted me in her stark white uniform and instructed me to lay down on my back on the bed. She proceeded to tell me I would just feel a slight sting as she stuck these sharp sticks into various positions over my head, lower stomach and feet. Then she told me to relax and left me on my own. I tried to turn my mind off and as they say, "just be in the moment." My mind was telling my body, "Relax Kellie, relax."

Stress is not a good thing at any time and most definitely not for anyone trying to fall pregnant. However, I am not sure I was overly stressed at the time. Yes, the IVF cycles were taking a toll on my body and my mind and the costs were starting to add up, but was I stressed? I was not sure. Anyway, I continued having acupuncture once a week for a few weeks but then stopped, as I felt like I was spending money and not getting any benefit. Maybe acupuncture worked for other women going through the same process, but for me, I was glad I at least gave it a try, even if it did not benefit me.

On our fourth IVF cycle with the same clinic, I had my egg retrieval on a Wednesday and was given the exciting news that eight eggs were collected, with four looking very healthy. After advice from the clinic professionals, Ian and I decided to take their advice and let four healthy embryos go to blastocyst. The definition of blastocyst is when an embryo has developed to the point of having two different cell components and a fluid cavity. These embryos develop in an IVF laboratory situation (or develop naturally in a body) and usually reach blastocyst by day five after fertilisation.

Blastocyst transfer from IVF can give a higher pregnancy success rate. We were told the laboratory staff would monitor the embryos closely in the laboratory and then only the healthier, more developed embryos would be transferred. We had the impression this was all new research; however, it did make sense to us and choosing to try blastocyst would give us a better chance of a successful pregnancy.

The following Saturday morning we received a call from the clinic stating three of the four embryos were developing as hoped. We looked at each other knowing we just had to get through to Monday. My parents were visiting over that time so on the Monday, while Ian was working in the yard with my dad, my mum came along to the clinic with me. It was just the routine embryo transfer and we were feeling really positive and excited with three good embryos waiting for us.

After arriving at the clinic, we were taken into a private waiting room. As the nurse came in I knew something was not right by the expression on her face. She gently explained that over the weekend the embryos had deteriorated and there was really no chance of a positive pregnancy result from any of them. The news was devastating and I could not stop crying or asking how it could have happened when everything had been going so well. I was in complete shock and could not get my head around it—I thought this was going to be the time it worked for us. How could it all go so wrong? What had I done to deserve this?

The nurses could not give me any straight answers as to why the embryos had deteriorated, which was extremely frustrating. In the end, the doctor decided to continue with the transfer procedure anyway. My mum told me afterwards she believed this was only done as I was very emotional and questioning the clinic. How the embryos could go from being so healthy to futile so quickly was something I could not understand at the time. I also could not get my head around the fact that my best chance at becoming pregnant had disappeared in only days.

The clinic offered us a discounted rate for our fifth IVF cycle, which Ian and I still believe they did as some form of compensation for a fault they were not prepared to admit to, like an electrical blackout; we experienced one at home that weekend so if the clinic also had an electrical failure, it would mean our embryos were not developing in the laboratory at the correct temperature. We turned down the offer for another IVF cycle as both agreed if we were going to do IVF again we

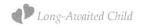

would have to try a different clinic. We were just too devastated and had lost our faith in this clinic. Plus, Ian and I knew we needed to have a little break from the routine of injections and clinic appointments that had become our life.

Chapter 3

OTHER OPTIONS

During the break between changing clinics, I started to look into other options of having a family. One evening I went along to a foster care seminar; Ian said I was clutching at straws and I believe he was right. I just yearned to have a baby to love so much. The foster care staff said we were a perfect couple to foster, even without knowing much about us; however, after much discussion, we decided to keep trying with IVF. The thought of the foster care system handing us a baby or child to care for and then possibly having that child removed from our care would just have been too heart-breaking for us at that time.

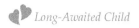

I commend anyone who is a foster parent on their strength and willingness to love a child whom they may have to give up. I know a few foster parents and it is not easy for them; however, I see how much love they have to give and I am so proud of what they do for their foster children. Even though foster care was not an option for Ian and me at the time, it may be an option for others, whether they already have had a family of their own or not. Those who choose this path, whether due to fertility issues or just because they have such big hearts and want to provide a loving home to a child in need, do so with the admiration of many, even if never expressed.

It is also not easy for foster parents, as the children they take in often struggle emotionally and physically from living in an unstable, unhealthy environment. Some foster parents even try to adopt their foster children, although this can be an understandably long and frustrating process. Fortunately, some states in Australia have introduced new legislations and reform packages such as "Safe Home for Life," in New South Wales. These aid to strengthen the child protection system so that every child has a safe home for life without going through a sometimes long and tedious adoption process. Another possibility foster parents may have

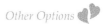

to be prepared for is their foster child(ren) returning to the natural birth parents.

The strength of these foster mums to let go of a child they have cared for and loved as if they were their own takes true strength. One foster care mum I know told me foster parents need to prepare themselves to have their hearts broken, and that's it's in no way a short-cut to the adoption process. At the time of taking on the responsibility to be a foster parent, prospective parents are legally informed that they may not get to keep a child should they later apply for adoption. It was then I knew fostering a child was not a task I could take on at that time, no matter how strong I had been in the past.

Everyone knows someone whose best friend's aunt's second cousin went to a particular IVF clinic and fell pregnant. After hearing from my best friend that her boss's wife had fallen pregnant after treatment at an IVF clinic in Brisbane, I got the particular doctor's information and went with it, especially since this doctor was known for a high success rate with producing IVF babies. Upon arriving at the clinic, I could tell that doctor was all business. I worried that I would be just another number and I knew I would not get to know the staff on a more personal level like at the

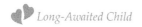

Nambour clinic. Still, I took a chance because I desperately wanted to be pregnant.

At my first appointment, I was given a schedule of hormones to inject and told when it should be done. When it was time for the egg retrieval surgery, Ian and I went to Brisbane and booked into a weekly stay at a hotel close to the doctor's clinic. We decided to stay from the day before the surgery until the embryo transfer five days later. This seemed an easier and more relaxed option than travelling back and forth from the Sunshine Coast, particularly since Ian also had some work in Brisbane. It was just a standard hotel room, nothing flashy, but it meant there would be nothing for me to do but relax, watch movies and order room service—the complete opposite of when I was at home pottering around the house and not resting like I was always instructed.

The night before the surgery we had dinner in the hotel restaurant. I hadn't gotten dressed up much of late so it was a nice change; at times, between the surgery and the embryo transfer, I was doing well if I worked up the care factor to even wash my hair. I remember sitting at the restaurant across from Ian feeling extremely sorry for myself. Up until that time, I did not think I had such strong emotions of "Why me?"

I was so down on myself, even when I kept trying to channel the part of me who was proud of my resilience. Yet at that time, I was struggling to find that part of me. My mind was telling me it was obviously all my fault and Ian should just go out and find himself a younger, more fertile woman. At one point over the years I even told him how I felt, to which he replied, "You cannot help who you fall in love with. Having children on top of that is just a bonus." How did I get so lucky to have him beside me?

Some days I felt like a robot: injections, ultrasounds, blood tests, surgery, transfers—I felt like shit and had received nothing for my troubles. Still, the next morning we went to the hospital for the procedure. No matter how many times I went through the surgery I always became quite teary beforehand. All sorts of crazy thoughts would enter my mind, like what if I never woke up from the surgery? Just in case, I would always call Mum and Dad the morning of the surgery to tell them I loved them.

This particular Brisbane hospital was a lot bigger than the small private hospital on the Sunshine Coast. It felt a bit like a production line; there was a queue of women waiting for exactly the same procedure as me. Why did I ever feel so alone when there were obviously

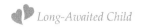

so many women going through all the same tiresome steps and procedures and hoping for the exact same outcome as me?

After the procedure, my bed was wheeled into a recovery room, which had about twelve other women all coming out of anaesthesia and recuperating after their procedure. This was far from quaint and personal. Overall, that was my worst experience with IVF. I was in a lot of discomfort after the surgery and was given morphine to ease the pain, which meant it was not the normal couple of hours until I was discharged from the hospital. There I was still in the recovery room drifting in and out of sleep for around six hours without Ian being allowed to sit by my bedside. He told me afterwards he was told to stay out in the waiting room. He was beside himself as he had not been given much information about why I was still in there, apart from that I had been experiencing some pain.

After I was eventually allowed to go back to the hotel with Ian I found a lovely surprise from him—a Tiffany & Co. bag with a gorgeous heart-shaped bangle inside. It was very sweet and a gift I will treasure forever. When I look at it now, it is a reminder of the challenges we have overcome and how far we have come as a couple.

Later that night, the extreme pain continued. I went to the toilet and could hardly sit down and when I did a large blood clot fell into the toilet. Due to my extended recovery time and the pain I had experienced in the hospital, the doctor had given Ian his direct mobile number to call should anything happen that night. Ian frantically called the doctor who said to take me immediately to the private hospital where I had the procedure earlier that day. There I was given more morphine and monitored for a few hours in the emergency room.

At that stage, I did not have private health coverage. The emergency room staff advised us that being transferred to a ward would cost us $5,000. Ian told me later he had felt pressured by the hospital administration staff into signing for me to be admitted; however, a lovely nurse took him aside and told him not to sign anything as the staff would still treat me the same in a privately screened room in the emergency ward. I am relieved he did not sign for that cost, as I was happy to stay in the emergency room on a bed. I was beyond caring about who saw me in agony, where I slept, or who got to witness my tears.

After being at the hospital for a few hours I was allowed back to the hotel but given strict rules to stay

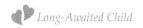

in bed until the embryo transfer. I could hardly walk due to the pain, so there was not much chance of me hitting the shops of Brisbane anyway.

As Ian was out during the day doing some contract work in Brisbane, my mum travelled down to stay with us at the hotel. She had been such a support through all of our ups and downs, so it was nice to have her there to keep me company. My doctor had been made aware of the outcome at the hospital and after two days asked me to come in for a check-up. He said with the embryos going to blastocyst, it still gave me another couple of days to heal and he felt confident I would be good as gold by then. I didn't.

Three days later and still in slight pain, I was back seeing the doctor for the embryo transfer. Mum knew the pain I had been in, which made us both doubt the embryo would implant, as who knew what the stress my body was going through with the bleeding and pain would do for the implantation. On the day of the transfer, one unhealthy embryo and two healthy embryos were transferred. There is a law in Australia, depending on your age, that determines how many embryos can be transferred during each IVF cycle. At my age, 35 at the time, it was two. I can understand the reasons behind that rule, however due to one of the embryos being unhealthy and likely to not implant, the doctor transferred the three. He then gave me a glass of brandy to drink, claiming it helps calm and relax the body. Two weeks later, we received another negative pregnancy test result.

However, like I said, different things work for different people. I have a new friend, Rachelle, who recently explained her wonderfully successful IVF story to me. She has two beautiful children now, a boy and a girl, both from IVF. Rachelle is one of the lucky ones who fell pregnant on her first IVF cycle; plus, she had some healthy embryos she was able to freeze for a few years before having some implanted and falling pregnant with her second child from the one IVF cycle. This does technically make her children twins even though they were born two years apart. In total she spent approximately $20,000, which included the storage of the frozen embryos. Her chosen IVF clinic was a large, well-known clinic in Sydney.

I cannot reiterate enough how amazing it is for so many people to have their own stories going on behind closed doors.

Chapter 4

TO ADOPT OR NOT TO ADOPT?

It was after the last harrowing IVF cycle that Ian and I decided to take a break from the emotional and expensive rollercoaster of in-vitro fertilisation. Our next step was to explore adoption as a possible option.

Attending a seminar in Brisbane being held by the Queensland government's Adoption Services, I was not sure Ian was as keen on the idea as me but he went along with me anyway. He could see I was trying to grab hold of any possibility of having a family of our own. I walked into the seminar looking all motherly

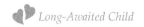

and responsible. I'm not sure how that looks but I remember wanting them to just think of me in that way, pick me, and hand me a baby immediately.

Unfortunately, the seminar was frustrating and not what I had been hoping it to be at all! We found it so infuriating to be informed it could be a seven-year wait until we were given a child, and during the time we were on the waitlist we were not allowed to continue with any IVF procedures. We struggled to understand the reasons behind this. If we had fallen pregnant naturally or by IVF, we would obviously just remove ourselves from the adoption waitlist.

This information was explained to us by a very young lady (and without sounding discriminatory) who I did not feel understood the desperation of the couples before her. On top of that, the father from the "golden family" of Queensland's Adoption Services was invited up on stage to talk about his adoption experience and how he and his wife had adopted two young children from overseas, as they awaited to receive their third child. They looked like they were on the lower side of their fifties, which also had me wondering what the cut off age was to adopt. It took a lot of control on my part to not stand up and yell out, "Back off, buddy! You have a family! Let someone else experience what it would feel like to have the opportunity to be a family!"

Instead, I walked away feeling very deflated but mostly angry that the Queensland and Australian adoption laws seemed so behind other countries'. We all see the magazine photos of celebrities in the USA with their adopted children; they seem to just have to say the word "adoption" and are given a baby to love in a heartbeat. I am sure it is not that easy for them, but it does seem to be a lot quicker and follows a more structured process than in Australia.

Ian and I were not in a position to go up against Queensland's Adoption Services with our opinions, so instead we went home where we quietly completed the first lot of paperwork for both intercountry and Queensland adoption. We were informed at the seminar that if we were prepared to take on a special needs child, we would almost be handed a child immediately. The financial toll of staying at home with a special needs child was not something we felt comfortable with or in the position to do. The reality of that is a big responsibility.

When Queensland's Adoption Services contacted us regarding our application, six months after our initial application submission, we were questioned numerous times on our lives and were, in the end, made to feel worthless. I am unsure why this occurred since both Ian and I had good jobs, no criminal records, owned a lovely home and had loving and supportive family and friends around us, some of whom had written glowing references about us as part of our application. We were even quietly harshly questioned over our residence and whether we were actually living in Queensland.

At one stage we received a letter to say we had not completed all required paperwork and without it our application would be dismissed. I contacted the adoption office immediately, as the paperwork had taken a lot of time to complete and I was positive it had all been sent and received. The lady I spoke with on the phone advised me she would look into it. I eventually received a call back to be informed the application paperwork had been found—someone in the office had incorrectly split it between the two adoption options we had applied for (intercountry and Queensland).

Slowly, we started to give up on our chances of adopting a child. The application process was mentally draining us, but more importantly the fact we could not try IVF again whilst waiting for the possibility we might be chosen to adopt a child did not feel like the right thing for us. Thus, we cancelled our adoption application. The seven-year waitlist was too long and we did not have the luxury of time. To this day, we still hear the stories and watch reports on television about adoption in Australia with disappointment; it is as if they have lost sight of the fact they are meant to be helping a child in need to become a part of a loving family.

So, our experience with Queensland's Adoption Services ended. Maybe the fact that, at the time, the law did not allow us to continue with an IVF cycle whilst going through the adoption application and waitlist made us give up on adoption too soon, but I was not ready to give up on the possibility of having a baby of our own through IVF. Fortunately, since late 2016, Queensland adoption laws have changed to allow couples undergoing fertility treatments to apply for adoption in Queensland.

However, that was my experience and I would not want to deter anyone from considering adopting if they think it might be an option for them. I recently had a conversation with a lovely mum, Chrissy, who has three adopted children through Queensland's Adoption Services. Hearing Chrissy's story, I realised she was very similar to me in the fact she did not necessarily believe she needed to be pregnant, she just knew she was desperate to be a mum. Chrissy and her husband went to an adoption seminar, just as Ian and I had, in Brisbane held by Queensland's Adoption Services. Chrissy was only 29 years old at the time and said she felt a little out of place as most of the other couples in the room appeared to be in their forties. Sitting there listening to the guest speakers though, she knew that was the place she was meant to be. Chrissy had had four IVF cycles over five years, with each cycle resulting in a pregnancy; however, she sadly miscarried each time. It was when she was driving home with her husband from the hospital after the fourth miscarriage that she heard an ad on the radio about the adoption seminar in Brisbane. She believed it was a sign, so she phoned to book their seats at the seminar straight away.

After attending the seminar, they completed the adoption paperwork and were contacted by Queensland's Adoption Services within three months to begin the application process. When talking with Chrissy about the application and interview processes, some of the words she used were stressful, offensive, and impersonal; however, she believes it is a process that works and all the information she was required to provide about their finances, relationship and health was warranted. An important point she made was these children are often already in foster care and growing attached to the foster parent. The adoption services want to be certain the adoptive parents are the right fit for each child, who is often just a baby, to ensure this is the final home the baby will be moved to.

Eighteen months after attending the seminar, Chrissy and her husband adopted their first child, a little girl who was eight months; which is old in adoption terms. It was one year later when they decided to adopt again, their second girl who was five months old. After another two years, Chrissy and her husband adopted a third child who was six months old. All three babies had previously been in foster care homes. Chrissy's story was so lovely to listen to and she believes her journey was meant to be, so much so that when she received the initial call that they had been selected to be the parents of a little girl, her body amazingly went through some symptoms over the next few days as if she was about to give birth and she started lactating. She said she was so shocked to receive the call, that without thinking she started writing the information given to her from the adoption agency on the wall in her house!

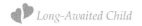

I asked Chrissy if she had any advice for anyone considering adoption and she said to just do it now — do not wait. Plus, be strong and be ready, which I interpreted in two ways: be ready for the interrogation, plus be ready for a baby. Chrissy mentioned applying to adopt only in Queensland rather than overseas seemed to be less of a wait. I am sure many others like the idea of adopting a child from overseas. Who would not want a gorgeous little baby to cuddle no matter where he or she was from? I was not aware of the difference in application times between adopting within Queensland compared to overseas; Chrissy was privy to this information and kept her application strictly to adopting a Queensland baby and it paid off beautifully for her.

What a wonderful feeling it must have been after the years of IVF and miscarriages and just wanting to be a mum to be handed her first child. Chrissy and her husband now have three girls (they have adopted over nine years) to tuck into bed each night. The girls are all aware they are adopted and Chrissy and her husband are open about not keeping anything a secret.

Chapter 5

NEW BEGINNINGS

For quite some time I had a calling to move to Perth, though I was not sure why as I had never been there before, and neither Ian nor I knew anyone who lived there. However, it was the following New Year's Eve when Ian and I were sitting on the deck of our newly built house enjoying a drink and talking about life when we made the decision we would go.

We started getting everything in order to make the move by the end of April that year. I was 36 and Ian was 40 and, after our fifth failed attempt at IVF and the options of foster care and adoption seeming like they were not for us, I felt I needed to escape the life we were currently living where decisions we made revolved around whether we were doing IVF at the time or whether I could possibly be pregnant. Sometimes I was just an emotional wreck. I felt like I was disappointing my friends and family by not being able to commit to any plans. They did not understand that doing IVF really controls all the choices you make, even some that might seem so simple.

On top of that, thanks to a very pregnant work colleague who I entrusted with my story, without knowing she was into oversharing whilst having a cigarette in the smoker's area (oh, the frustrations!), the word got around at work of my fertility struggle. With a large office full of young women, most of the time it was a lot of fun and I was always excited for a colleague when she made the exciting announcement she was expecting. It became harder when although I had not given anyone any reason to think it would upset me if they told me they were pregnant, they took it upon themselves to assume I would be. I hated the sympathy and I didn't want a pity party. I loved my job, our new home and where we lived but I had to get away!

The move to Perth was exciting. It was just Ian and I along with all the belongings we could fit into our 4WD. Everything else had been put in storage, along with my disappointment of being unsuccessful in IVF. We had no jobs to go to, nowhere to live and no friends to help out—it was just us. It kind of felt like we were starting from scratch and leaving all our troubles back in Queensland. I loved every minute of it! We made a holiday out of driving across the country stopping, at various towns and sights we had always been interested in visiting. Our life started to feel fun and easy again. We had lots of laughs along the way and made some lovely memories together. Once in Perth we both soon found jobs and an apartment right in the city. I loved so much about our fresh start in Perth and knew deep down this move had been the right decision.

After being in Perth for a while and getting our lives set up here, Ian and I started having conversations about possibly looking into international surrogacy as an option. We watched a story on *60 Minutes* some years earlier in which two gay Australian men in a relationship had used an egg donor and surrogate from overseas. It was just so unheard of at the time. Ian and I both remember being wowed by the story the two men told. We feel indebted to those two guys

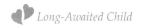

for sharing their story; if we had not seen it, we may never have known overseas surrogacy was an option for us.

Ian is the researcher in our relationship. He would explore all the big questions in our life and would then give me the summary of information I needed to know so we could make a decision together. For me it was perfect, as sitting at a computer searching for answers did nothing for me. In this case, deciding to look further into international surrogacy possibly in India or even Thailand, Ian started his researching. After looking into the surrogacy laws of both countries, we decided we might choose India. After all, they were at the forefront of intercountry surrogacy.

At the time, Thailand did not have any laws in place regulating surrogacy for foreign couples, which meant if the surrogate mother decided she wanted to keep the baby she could and she was not legally bound to hand the child over. I could not imagine going through all of the processes and costs to then have the surrogate mother not give us our baby. It would be frustrating and completely devastating. Also, we had heard the stories from Thailand where a surrogate mother had held the intended parents ransom and would not allow the baby to be taken away unless the intended parents paid her more money. On the other hand, India's surrogacy laws were based on strict contractual laws signed by both the surrogate mother, her husband, and the intended parents. For these reasons, it was a no-brainer for us; India was where we would go for a surrogate.

When researching, we (well, Ian) found numerous surrogacy clinics located around India. On 4th September 2011, we made our first initial enquiries with clinics in both Mumbai and New Delhi. We received email responses from both the next day outlining all services available along with the costs. Their fee programs were very straightforward in what each service included and the required time to send each progressive payment. After researching and reading the information in the emails from the clinics, we decided to go with the clinic in New Delhi as it had a good success rate plus a well-known doctor in the industry who owned and ran the clinic. Ian really decided on this clinic and I was happy to let him, as I could not make a decision with too many what-ifs going around in my head.

Over the next few months, we kept our communication up with two female staff members of the clinic who were located in Australia. They had been

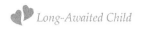

through the same processes to have their own families and afterwards became employed by the clinic to help any Australians through the process all the way up to the point of collecting your child in India. I had a LOT of questions. It really felt like the unknown. We did not personally know anyone who had been down this path before us.

A short time after Christmas, my parents came to visit us in Perth. I loved Perth and I was proud of my new city. One day I was showing them around the sights of the city when I started to have some bleeding followed by a large blood clot. That cut short our day of exploring the city very quickly. The following day I was able to see a doctor who arranged for some tests, which confirmed I had cysts on my uterus and I needed surgery to have them removed, preferably as soon as possible. He said they were most likely not cancerous but if not removed they could become cancerous. The thought had not even crossed my mind until he said that dreaded "C" word. Thankfully, he was right, and they were not.

During one of my pre-surgery appointments, the gynaecologist informed me that with these cysts in my uterus, it was highly unlikely I would have ever fallen pregnant, but he could not say how long the cysts had been there. This bit of information absolutely crushed me. My mind went into an overdrive of questions. Were they there the whole time we were paying for and going through expensive IVF procedures in Queensland? Had I just never had medical professionals experienced enough to discover the cysts? Had they only formed after the traumatic IVF experience in Brisbane? Had I just wasted years of my life, not to mention money? So many questions, to which, once again, I would never know the answers. I was so irate this curve ball had been thrown in the mix to add to everything else we had been through.

To remove the cysts from my uterus, the surgery involved going through my body three ways: a "key-hole" through my belly button, an incision through my stomach, and through the vagina. It took a few weeks for my body to recover from the surgery since I was in a lot of pain from the surgeon having to cut my stomach muscle.

Once I was back to my old self again, and all the cysts were removed, Ian wanted to continue looking further into international surrogacy; however, with the cysts now gone I felt like I owed it to myself to have one more shot at IVF. What if my failures to conceive were due to the cysts? I needed to explore this possibility so, once again, I endured hormone injections and made up excuses at work as to why I was late or had to leave early for regular ultrasounds and blood tests, not to mention my emotions were all over the place. Some mornings before my work day had even started I had injected needles into my stomach and been for blood tests and scans. It was hard at times to keep my emotions in check when dealing with demanding hotel guests.

During the dreaded two-week wait for the pregnancy test result, I knew inside it hadn't worked. I guess over time we get to know our bodies quite well; at the time, I just knew we were not pregnant. Ian and I had already decided if we had another negative result, we would definitely contact the clinic we had chosen in New Delhi to start planning the surrogacy option. Even though the thought of another negative result was devastating for me, just knowing we had a Plan B (or was it Plan E?) up our sleeves allowed me to get through the two-week wait a lot easier.

Not long after we had received the negative pregnancy test result, I was contacted by the Perth IVF clinic to see if I was interested in a clinical trial. There had started to be some research in the industry suggesting some females might have a very high immune system in which their body would fight off the transferred embryo as a "foreign" object, just like it would with the flu virus. This did make some sense, as I was never ill. Or, if I ever did become ill, what would take a normal person weeks to fight off would take me one day. The industry had also started a trial for testing and a new drug to go along with this research. I was offered to go on the trial, which would mean a free IVF cycle. It was tempting, knowing the costs involved with IVF, which I would not have to pay; however, I could not bring myself to go through another cycle. I don't regret this decision. My body was done with the hormone injecting, and I had been through enough emotional turmoil. Anyway, there was no guarantee being on the trial drugs would help with my IVF success.

IVF Australia and Queensland Fertility Group have information on their websites about Natural Killer (NK) Cell Testing (the source of the experiment) and it appears tests are now being conducted on patients who have had a continuous record of miscarriages or non-stop unsuccessful IVF cycles. They are both very interesting reads and something I would have looked into further had it been around when I was in the first few years of IVF.

Chapter 6

INTERNATIONAL SURROGACY PROGRAM

In May 2012, I sent an email to the clinic in India advising them of our extreme interest in their services and asked what steps we needed to take to get the process up and running. We still had so many questions regarding timeframes and egg donors

I did consider the idea of asking my sister, Jodie, to be our surrogate in Australia and I know if I had she would not have hesitated. At the time, Australian laws for surrogacy were quite strict, having to prove why we were in need of a surrogate and why I was not able to carry a baby naturally. It felt like the red tape we would have to go through would once again lengthen the process for us. In the end, this did not feel like it was the best option for us. I am now so thankful we didn't go down that path, as I think there would always be that part of me that would feel insecure when my sister was around my child. I know my sister would not make me feel that way, but I would always be watching to see if there was some hidden bond between her and my baby that would be stronger than my bond with my baby. If I had a baby of my own, I did not want to question our love or our bond.

We informed the clinic we were interested in the gestational surrogacy program, an arrangement in which a woman, the gestational surrogate, carries and delivers a baby for another person. The egg comes from the intended mother or, in our case, an egg donor, and not the surrogate herself. The sperm would come from the intended father, Ian.

The DNA testing requirements state for international clients they cannot use both an egg and a sperm donor, or donor embryos with surrogacy, as a genetic link between baby and at least one parent is required by the embassies of most countries to grant citizenship and a passport to the baby. A genetic link is established through DNA testing of one parent and baby. This is a mandatory requirement for citizens of most countries.

Initially we were going to go down the path of using my eggs and Ian's sperm. I was told I could have had the hormones provided to me in Australia and the surgery for egg retrieval in India; however, I feared a small quantity or poorer quality of eggs would not be retrieved during surgery. This seemed to be what happened in the past with me. Plus, there was a lot of miscommunication as to whether this was legal. I was handed a lot of different opinions from the clinic and the ladies working for them in Australia and I was not sure what to believe. In the end, Ian and I decided that, due to the costs of international surrogacy, this was most likely going to be our one and only shot of trying to fall pregnant using a surrogate, so we had to go with the option that would best give us our chance of a positive outcome, and if that meant using a donor egg then that was what we had to do.

Not being my child's biological mother was not something I had thought much about until now and it was something I had to learn to accept very quickly. I did, at times, question whether I would love this child as much compared to a child being biologically mine, as I didn't already have children of my own to understand the type of love you have for your child. I am definitely an over-thinker. Before now I always believed I just wanted to be a mum and was not really concerned how I had or was given this child, but here I was having to face my reality that my possible only chance of having a child was for it not to be biologically mine.

One afternoon when out walking with a friend, she gave me the best answer possible to my concerns and one I will never forget. She said to me, "You have a stepdad who you call Dad and who looks at you as one of his own and loves you because you are a part of your mother, the woman he loves. Then why would this be any different when the baby would biologically be Ian's?" This simple reminder of my life was the best advice and exactly what I needed to hear to quash any doubts in my head. Yes, there is a man who married my mum when I was five years old whom I have called Dad ever since. And yes, even though I am not biologically his daughter, I know he loves me as his very own, as I look at him and love him as my dad.

The process for international surrogacy in India was very straightforward—well, when I look back, it felt straightforward compared to the back and forth routine at the IVF clinics. Our surrogacy clinic was very prompt with their replies. Once we had confirmed we would like to go ahead with the program, they replied there was no wait as they had egg donors and surrogates always ready to go. We initially had to provide the clinic with some test results that were less than 12 months old from my IVF procedures, Ian's semen analysis as well as if either of us already had children (which we did not). The doctor from our clinic in New Delhi would then review all our information and advise us of the best way to proceed.

The clinic emailed us a list of possible egg donors to choose from, all listed by an ID number. We were not given much information on the donors apart from a few basics: eye colour, height, region she was from, partial education information and a photo. We chose someone who was the same height as me, but that is where our similarities in appearances ended. You see, I have blonde hair and blue eyes, the opposite end of the scale to someone with Indian heritage. We were informed the further south in India the woman lived, the darker the skin. For this reason, we also chose someone from the north so the child would have skin on the lighter side of olive. The donor is never the

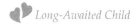

same person as the surrogate mother to ensure there is less of a chance of a bond forming between the surrogate mother and the baby. We went back to the clinic with a few donor numbers and were advised our first choice was available.

It is funny how they say things can happen for a reason and in our case, this seemed to be true. At the time, international surrogacy was not legal in all states of Australia, with Queensland being one of the states that deemed it illegal; however, in Western Australia it was legal. If we had not moved to Perth, we may never have looked any further into this process, but there we were taking another step towards becoming parents thanks to my inner need to move to Perth.

Overall, after completing the paperwork, including Ian's semen test result, selecting a donor, obtaining our visas to enter India, and having our annual leave time from work, we were on our way. We also provided the clinic with our flight and accommodation details as they would have a driver meet us at the airport to take us to our hotel. Our first deposit, which was one of many extremely large payments, was made at that time also.

One thing we also had to do, which took us by

surprise but at the same time was understandable, was name two people in Australia who would be responsible for collecting our baby should we not return ourselves. Sure, I get this could be the case, if for example we were involved in an accident of some sort. Or sadly, as has apparently happened in the past, if a couple separates and neither wants the child. The thought breaks my heart. I could not imagine the lengths a couple would endure to have a child only to change their mind at the last minute.

For me, I was so grateful to know I had the right partner for me along this journey. Our hopes and plans for a child were, once again, underway and I tell you Ian and I could not be any happier.

Chapter 7

INDIA

On 31st July 2012, we flew out of Perth for India. I would have to say the flight from Singapore to India was possibly the worst flight of my life. I had booked Qantas, not knowing the flight from Perth to Singapore would be on a Qantas plane, but from Singapore to New Delhi we would be put on the Indian airline Jet Airways.

I remember sitting in my seat squashed between Ian and some stranger thinking, "What am I doing to us and putting us through?" The food was horrible and the passengers were rude and pushy. On top of that, there seemed to be no concern for safety from the

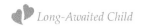

passengers or even the crew at times. I am sure at one stage I even contemplated opening the emergency exit door and jumping out. However, eighteen hours after leaving Perth we finally made it to New Delhi, India in one piece.

After collecting our bags and finding our driver, we went straight to our hotel. We were exhausted and after that long, unenjoyable flight we needed a long, hot shower and sleep. We had booked a five-star hotel, The Imperial, on Connaught Place, Janpath, New Delhi, which, according to Ian's research, was about a 15-minute drive to either the clinic or hospital. We chose this hotel not just because it looked amazing, but more importantly because it appeared safe with very strict security. The building was set back from the street with lovely gardens to separate the hotel from the street and had thick, high concrete fences with barbed-wire stretched out on top. There were guards at the gates with rifles checking the boot and glove compartment of any vehicle entering the hotel grounds before the driver was given permission to drive in. It may sound more like a prison but once inside the concrete walls surrounding the perimeter of the hotel it was stunning and, most importantly, we felt safe there.

The following day after arriving in New Delhi, we

took a taxi from our hotel for our first appointment at our chosen clinic. The hotel concierge called us a taxi from the long line of taxis ready to take the guests to their chosen sightseeing destinations for the day. Our driver pulled up in a beat-up old car, but that was ok with us as we were just happy to be there. Also, he was so honest and friendly, we could not help but like him instantly. His English was basic but he seemed to know his way around the hectic, large city so that was the main thing.

The traffic in New Delhi was outrageous. I am not sure why they even had designated lanes, as the drivers did what they wanted, yet no one appeared to show any signs of road rage; they just gently beeped their way through.

It was our first trip to India and we did not know what to expect. The friendliness of the locals was a welcoming surprise. If you have been to New Delhi or any of the large cities in India you would know what I mean when I say the streets are overcrowded, dirty, and polluted. New Delhi has a population of over 22 million people, so we did expect it to be busy, but I do not think you can fully comprehend the life and living conditions until you see it for yourself. It constantly amazed me how the people appeared so happy with so little. I was not sure where they washed their clothes as many lived in makeshift buildings on the side of the road yet their clothes were so clean and white. Outside our surrogacy clinic, the streets were congested and noisy and there were power lines overhead running in every direction, people walking, begging or selling their wares, and dogs aimlessly roaming around. None of this mattered to us, as when we arrived at the clinic, it was like stepping into a familiar office in Australia—they were really friendly and the office was modern, clean, immaculate, and air-conditioned.

Whilst in the waiting room, I met a new mum from Australia who was there with her newborn baby to say her final goodbyes to their surrogate mother. Chatting with this lady and hearing her story gave me hope that maybe this could work for us as well. I also recall her telling me when she was returning to Australia she was going on the trial drug for females with a high immune system. I wish I had taken her details as I would love to know how her story continued.

Ian and I then met the senior doctor who owned the surrogacy business along with her administration team who we had been dealing with via email. We were given instructions that the following day we would be required to meet the lawyer back at the clinic to sign contractual paperwork. We were also informed when Ian would be required to provide his semen sample at the hospital. We were offered a driver, at an additional cost, during our stay if needed; however, we decided we would continue to use the driver we had that morning. He had been sincere and outgoing and it was obvious he needed the work and money to provide for his family.

That meeting was the first of many surreal moments for us. After the appointment, we went back to our hotel without even going to our room; instead, we headed to the hotel bar to get a very much-needed alcoholic beverage. We sat out in the stunning hotel gardens enjoying a drink and trying to calm our minds whilst listening to the sounds of New Delhi—mostly the continuous beeping of car horns. That afternoon of drinks at the hotel bar was similar to many others on the overwhelming days that followed.

Our second appointment the next day was a meeting with the lawyer at the clinic to sign a 36-page confidentiality document. We were not offered the opportunity to seek a lawyer for ourselves, however the lawyer employed by the clinic was fair to both parties and ensured the document was read and understood fully. This document was our Gestational Surrogacy

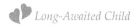

Agreement enforced by the National Capital Territory of Delhi. There were many points covered in this contract, including the surrogate not having claim over the child. It also stated the baby would genetically belong to the intended parents, being both Ian and myself.

We allowed the clinic to select our surrogate for us. The Indian government had introduced a law stating surrogates had to be married with children of their own. Our surrogate mother, Manu, had a husband and a five-year-old son and was from a village a few hours away from New Delhi. Unfortunately, that was pretty much all the information we were given on Manu. Our surrogate and her husband visited the clinic at a different time than us to sign the contract.

There was the option to have two surrogates with embryos transferred to each of them at the same time for an extra cost. This, of course, would increase the success rate of a pregnancy; however, this suggestion did boggle our minds when contemplating if embryos were implanted in both women, the possibility of several multiples could occur. We graciously declined this offer.

The day Ian was to provide his sperm sample at the hospital, we called our driver to take us there. Amongst all of the chaotic traffic, our driver suddenly stopped at a roundabout, got out of his car, collected birdseed and water from the car boot, and fed the pigeons on the traffic islands. To us, this was very bizarre, however, to him it was part of his every day routine, and the drivers of the cars stuck behind him at the roundabout just beeped their horns and moved into another lane. We later looked into this and it is a ritual performed by many local people who believe doing this is their way of seeking a stairway to Heaven. I love witnessing new experiences and customs when visiting another country.

Before leaving for India, we had read a few stories on social media about how these poor Indian women, who were prepared to be surrogates, were being taken advantage of and the inhumane way they were used. However, these accusations were made by one of many people who did not, and possibly still do not, understand the full story of surrogacy in India. The decision for the woman to become a surrogate is completely her own. Additionally, the money Manu would earn by being our surrogate was equivalent to her husband's salary over ten years; it would provide her and her family with the finances to buy a family home and give her son a proper education.

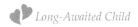

Another rule of the clinic was the surrogates, along with their husband and children, were able to stay in a house provided by the clinic. This was to ensure a doctor was always on hand and the surrogate was well cared for with her diet and rest. The clinic often said the health of the surrogate mums was their first priority. It was a nice relief to know they were well cared for and treated with respect and dignity.

I understand the emotions our surrogate, carrying another couple's baby for nine months, would possibly endure knowing at birth the child would be taken away from her and she would never again see the child she gracefully carried. Knowing if I was in her situation and carrying a child for someone else meant providing a better life for my family, I would do exactly the same thing. Even more so after seeing the living conditions of so many Indian families.

Overall, we spent ten days in New Delhi. Ian and I were often amazed by how India, a developing country, has hospitals and clinics that were so clean and run so efficiently and how couples from all over the world were seeking Indian medical professionals to help them have a baby. It was so exciting to look through the window of the nursery to see the babies. As I gazed at the newborn faces of children swaddled in blankets, I could not help but think how, maybe, one day, our baby would be there and we would be standing at the door ready to enter and meet him or her for the first time.

Even prior to our trip to India, it had never been on our bucket list of destinations to travel to; however, it really is an amazing country and one I now hold very close to my heart. The people are so beautiful and kind. Mostly, our stay was about completing paperwork and procedures, though we did have a few free days. On one day we decided to have a hotel driver take us up to see the Taj Mahal—a must-see attraction and magnificent structure in India. My main memory of that day was how hot it was—one of the hottest days in my life. It was, after all, the middle of an Indian summer.

To be honest, at that stage we did not even know if we would ever be returning to India. Yes, we would if our surrogate did become pregnant; however, if surrogacy did not work the first time, we were not sure there would be a second chance with the costs involved. Unfortunately, we were not permitted to meet our egg donor, but we do have her photo. Meeting our surrogate, Manu, during the trip did not occur either. So, whilst all these procedures were being done at the hospital, Ian and I were back at the hotel swimming in the pool and having conversations of "What if this worked?" Just imagining in approximately nine months we could be back in India to meet our baby brought the biggest smiles to our faces. This was such an amazing and unforgettable experience to be having together. After all the paperwork had been completed, our egg donor had been through the egg retrieval procedure, and our surrogate had the embryo transfer procedure, it was time for us to head back to Australia.

When I initially booked our flights, I had the idea we would have a stopover at Singapore, a lovely destination, for a short holiday before returning home and to work. I had booked our accommodation at the Rendezvous Hotel not far from the shopping strip, Orchard Road, as it was the hotel chain I was working for at the time and nothing beats staff rates. It was not my best idea, as Ian and I tried to do the tourist thing, but our minds were not in the right headspace. We did manage to venture out a few times and went to the famous Singapore Zoo for breakfast with the baboons, over to Sentosa Island and Marina Bay Sands Complex, and, of course, a spot of shopping, but most of the time we just were not feeling the tourist vibe.

I mainly just wanted to be back at the hotel staring at our laptop in hopes an email would come through from the clinic as to how our surrogate, Manu, was doing. Even though I knew we still had to go through the two-week wait before a pregnancy test would even be done, I was eager for some form of email indicating she was pregnant. We would email the clinic asking how Manu was doing and they would reply saying she was well and resting. Apart from that, there really was no information to be passed onto us at that point. It was a waiting game and we just had to sit tight.

Chapter 8

COULD WE BE PREGNANT?

Back in Australia, we settled into our normal routine of work, hanging out with friends, daily life, etc., but we were also checking our emails every possible moment for updates on Manu. We were informed all communication would be via email, unless it was really good news or, sadly, very bad news, which would then entail a phone call from the head doctor.

Wednesday, 22nd August 2013 was the day we were to receive the email on Manu's pregnancy test results and it was like any normal day for me. We had only been home from our time in Singapore for about one week. I was at work and Ian was at home. Ian worked on a four-week away, one-week home roster so it was nice to have him at home for a little longer as we waited on the pregnancy test result. Whilst at work that afternoon, I noticed on my personal email account inbox an email from our clinic in New Delhi, but I did not dare open it. What if it was bad news in the form of a negative pregnancy test and I became a blubbering mess at work? What if it was good news and Manu was pregnant? I would want to be home to share that moment with Ian. We had not yet had the conversation about what we would do if this did not work the first time around, yet we had already decided if we were to have a baby, we would be happy with just the one and would be a family of three.

I raced home with my heart in my mouth. When I got there, I had to get Ian to open the email—I could not look. He read it out: "CONGRATULATIONS! You are now pregnant!"

I think we had a moment of looking stunned before we both burst into tears. After hugging each other, I ran around our apartment like a lunatic. I could not believe it was finally happening for us. In that one moment of reading that email, we knew our lives were going to be changed forever. It was no longer going to just be the two of us. We were *finally* going to have the family we so much desired.

After absorbing the news and calming down a bit, we rang our families and friends who knew about our surrogacy journey in India. Everyone was so emotional and excited for us and, I think, they were a little shocked also that after everything we had been through it had actually worked on the first attempt. Ian and I hardly slept that night. After all the years of trying and not giving up, it looked like our dream to be parents was going to come true. Apart from those who knew, we kept this beautiful little secret to ourselves for quite some time, as it was in the early days of the pregnancy and there was still the chance so much could go wrong.

The next day I was able to phone the clinic for more information. I was advised Manu was well and four embryos had been implanted with one splitting so that meant there was a possible chance of five babies — three individual and a set of identical twins. Unlike Australia that has strict rules on the number of embryos transferred, in India the doctor can transfer as many as he or she feels right. This can be a good thing for a higher success rate; however, it can also be a downside if all of the embryos are taken without any others to try again

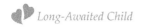

at a later stage, or there could be multiples. Sure, we wanted a family, but we would not have been prepared for *five* newborns!

The clinic reminded me their first priority was the health of the surrogate mother, so in this case after a couple of weeks of watching the growth and development of the embryos, they would be performing a "selective reduction" in which, depending on the health of each embryo, they would reduce the number down to two, keeping the two healthiest embryos. I completely understood the reasons behind the procedure though the information devastated me. I could not believe after all we had been through to have a baby, the "selective reduction" was really another term for a termination or abortion. Plus, during this procedure there was the risk of losing all five embryos. One minute we were elated over Manu being pregnant with our babies, the next we were in complete panic at the thought of losing them all.

Initially, we were advised of all the payment conditions for which invoices would be sent out over the term of the pregnancy. Being aware of all costs from the beginning, the only deterrent was that each time something unplanned happened, like the procedure for the selective reduction, we were emailed another invoice.

We were dumbfounded by how quickly the clinic sent these invoices to us and how expediently they wanted the payment to be made. It felt a bit daunting at times as I would go to the bank to make an international transfer for thousands of dollars at a time to a company in another country who we were entrusting to do the right thing by us.

Not long after we had paid for the selective reduction procedure, the clinic informed us the reduction had happened naturally and we were left with two thriving embryos. I am not sure if this was the truth, but I did not question the clinic over it or ask for our money back for the procedure—I did not want to talk about it and just preferred to believe the information was the honest truth. The loss of the other three embryos, identical twins from the split embryo and one individual, hit us harder than expected. Nature really can amaze you and crush you at the same time. It was sad thinking of the possible babies that could have been. So, there we were, hoping for one baby and it actually looked like we were going to have two—and just like that, we were ecstatic again.

The nine months Manu was pregnant with our babies were really a rollercoaster of highs and lows, although in some ways it was easier than dealing with

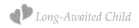

the medical appointments, blood tests and emotions of IVF. I got on with my work—canoe outrigging, which I loved—and life with Ian who was away for weeks at a time and then home again for a week, but in the back of my mind I was constantly thinking of Manu and our babies.

It was easier for Ian, without sounding like he has no emotions; he made himself think of the whole thing as a business transaction. I think for him it was his way of protecting himself in the event of things souring or the possible loss of the babies. Whereas for me, even though I had not yet met Manu, I felt some form of bond with her. Maybe it was just a part of being female that we had a strong womanly bond, along with my desperation for this opportunity to work. I was constantly emailing the clinic to check on Manu and sending over gifts for her. The clinic once told me I was the nicest mother-to-be to her surrogate. That was nice to know, but to me, Manu was prepared to give me the world and the small gestures I made were nothing in comparison.

Six months after returning from India, there was a change to the international surrogacy laws in India. When we first enquired, the law was any couple could enter a surrogacy agreement providing they had been in a relationship for a minimum of two years, though this did not necessarily have to be a marriage; hence, the reason international surrogacy in India was an option for same sex couples wanting to have a family. The law changes at the time stated any couple entering an agreement had to be married for a minimum of two years. Thankfully, as our surrogate was already pregnant, this change in law did not apply to us. At that stage in our lives, Ian and I had been in a de facto relationship for nine years but we had never married. I think once we decided to try for a baby, with all that followed, it took over our life and being married did not become as important. We are still not married today. If this had been the law back when we had initially enquired, I am not sure if we would have rushed out to marry and wait the two years to then apply. Our age was always a concerning factor for us and by then we may just have felt too old. Yet, thanks to our pregnancy occurring before the alteration in the law, we avoided that hurdle—at least we had one issue in our favour.

During the months Manu was pregnant with our twins, most of the time we tried best we could to get on with our lives, though there were many scary moments when Manu was in the hospital. We were always told by the clinic not to worry, but that is easier said than

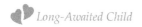

done. We had a lady, a stranger really, in another country carrying our babies and I had no control over how she was feeling or doing. It was hard not to worry.

The October prior to our twins being born my parents were on a caravanning trip; at the time they were in Exmouth, Western Australia, I flew up to spend a week with them. My mum later told me she could not believe how unhealthy I looked when I got off the plane; the stress must have really been taking a toll on my body and skin. Luckily, after a week of relaxing, swimming in the gorgeous, clear waters of Coral Bay, enjoying a nightly glass of wine with my parents, and having my mum cook healthy dinners of fish and salad, I felt like a new person going back to Perth. The time away was just what I needed to refocus and get my mind prepared for the next few months of waiting.

In November, I had a few of my school friends from Hervey Bay come to visit. It was hard to keep my amazing secret a secret. Two of my friends already had four children of their own and the other one had five children. Surely, they would not understand the struggles I had endured. I had a great time with them visiting and it was a good distraction from the reality of my life.

* * * *

Even though we had known of the upcoming birth of our babies since August, I still had not told anyone at work I was going to be a mummy. This was not easy to do as some of my work colleagues were also my friends and I was bursting at the seams to tell them. I wanted to hold off for as long as I could, which without a growing baby bump was a lot easier to do.

I had the loveliest manager at work and was excited to tell him but I waited until after the New Year, as that was only four or so months until our babies were due. One particular morning when I knew I just could not keep my secret in any longer, I rang my manager to arrange a meeting with him. I had previously told him in conversation, well before my first visit to India, that Ian and I were not sure if we wanted children—my normal response, which I had gotten very good at saying to cover up the embarrassment I felt for not being able to have children of my own. We sat down and I told him of our Indian surrogacy story to date. Reactions like his are ones I will never forget; he was genuinely so excited for us and wanted all the details. After telling my manager, I also informed my hotel General Manager and my team. Everyone was shocked, as they had no idea, but more importantly, they were all thrilled for us. It really was very lovely to

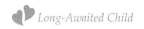

have so much excitement and support around me.

Towards the end of the pregnancy, Manu was in and out of hospital quite often. I was stressed every time I was sent an email, along with another invoice for her hospital stay. I often called the clinic after receiving these emails, but they informed me not to worry too much about Manu and that they had to take extra good care of the surrogate mother to ensure her health is the main priority. In other words, if I was pregnant myself back in Australia and not well, my doctor may insist on bed rest at home; however as the health of the surrogate mother is the main priority to them, they have to admit her to hospital.

There have been suggestions and opinions on some blogs how this is a way for the clinic to get more money out of the intended parents, as each hospital visit meant another invoice requesting payment for the surrogate's hospital stay. I do not know if there is even a slight bit of truth to this, but I like to believe there isn't and they were just taking the best care of our surrogate. Anyway, what option did we have except to continue to pay the invoices? There really was no point in looking for negative opinions. Manu was carrying our babies and no one was going to burst this bubble for us.

In the beginning of March, as time grew closer to our arrival date, my lovely friends planned a baby shower for me. Even three of my very close friends flew over from the East Coast for the weekend, which really meant the world to me. It was not your normal baby shower where everyone sits around playing games and eating cupcakes with a very pregnant mother-to-be. In the afternoon we were all frocked up and ready to celebrate. My friend hosting the party for me had done an amazing job of decorating with all the cute baby things you would normally see at a baby shower. Nevertheless, the drink of choice for the afternoon was champagne which I drank from the moment of arriving at my friend's house and continued to do so the duration of the party. So, as I was saying, not your average baby shower. To this day, I get a little bit of enjoyment when I say to people, unaware of my situation, that I was a little drunk at my baby shower — their shocked faces are priceless. I know deep down on the day I was feeling overwhelmed, anxious, plus scared (with Manu being in hospital again and the due date nearing). I guess I had one of those moments where I drank to cover up how I was really feeling on the inside, and even though I had plenty of laughs that afternoon with my friends my thoughts were never far from Manu and my babies. My friends and work

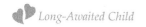

colleagues were extremely generous with their gifts and I was overwhelmed by how kind they all were. It really was an amazing and fun day.

Manu's 40 week mark was 1st May, however, the medical team at the hospital advised us they would be delivering our babies by caesarean on 10th April. Our flights were booked to arrive a few days prior. Everything was starting to become very real.

We did not know the sex of our little twins and were informed there was a law in India stating the sex of babies cannot be revealed prior to birth. We did not mind; all we knew was there were two babies that were not identical that would be our children. We would have been happy for one happy, healthy baby, but there we were getting two (for the price of one).

We had started to think of names to prepare for scenarios of either two boys or two girls or one of each. Ian and I both love holidaying in Hawaii so one day when Ian was looking up names he came across a Hawaiian boy's name, Bane, which means long-awaited child. We both instantly fell in love with the name and meaning and knew if we were having a boy his name would be Bane. We threw around ideas of a few other boy and girl names, though nothing

else grabbed us at the time. Imagine, years of trying naturally and then round after round of IVF all
unsuccessfully producing a baby for us and now we
were contemplating the *names* of our *children*!

Chapter 9

OUR BABIES' ARRIVAL

Wednesday, 13th March 2013, was a normal day at work. Ian was once again home, so after work we went out for dinner (something we used to do a lot when he was home and prior to having children). They were the days of being DINKS—double income no kids. It was a warm night so we walked to our favourite restaurant near our home in the city area of Perth. It was a lovely night with delicious food, a few drinks, and, as always, our conversation revolved around our babies and how we could not believe we were going to be parents soon. My thoughts were often of Manu and that night was no exception. She had been admitted again to the hospital a few days prior; I had received an email that day from the clinic advising she was doing well and not to worry. The staff knew me by that point and understood how much I worried about Manu and our babies so I think we received more updates than any other parents-to-be.

Later that night at 10.25 pm, Ian and I were just getting into bed when my phone rang. From the number on the display I could tell the call was coming from India. In total panic, I yelled out to Ian, "It is India!" It flashed into my mind how we were told we would only receive a call when it was either very good or very bad news. From the email I had received earlier, all were doing fine so why was I receiving this call? Manu was only 33 weeks pregnant so surely our babies had not come early. My heart was racing. Did this call mean it was going to be bad news?

I answered and a doctor from the clinic said, "Hello, Kellie. Congratulations, you have a little boy and a little girl."

I can still clearly remember in my mind every word he said in his Indian accent. I started crying. Ian's face exhibited dread, as he had not heard the doctor and only saw me crying. I hung up the phone and told Ian our babies were born and we had a little boy and a little girl. It was such an emotional moment for us. Eight years of putting so much on hold had almost come to an end. Now, we were actually going to have the family we had been wanting for so long. I was going to be a mummy to two little humans. I was no longer going to be the lady walking down the street whose heart would break when she saw a mum push her babies in a stroller or the mum feeding her baby in a café. *I* was going to be part of an amazing group of women. *I was a mummy.*

Before I had hung up the phone, I had been given the number for the doctor who had delivered our babies and I was able to call him. He informed me Manu and both babies were doing well. Once again, we phoned our family and friends and did not care that the time difference meant it was almost one in the morning in Queensland. We knew everyone would want to know. Certain family and friends had taken the journey with us so how could we not let them know straight away?

Our twin babies had been born at 33 weeks. Our baby boy, Bane, had weighed 1.87 kilograms (4.12

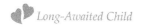

pounds) and our little girl 2.04 kilograms (4.49 pounds). They were tiny but doing well.

So, there I was at 39 years old and a new mummy to two gorgeous babies. As planned, we named our son Bane with the middle name Max after my (step) dad and for our little daughter we had chosen the Hindi name Daya, which means compassion, with the middle name Poppy as I thought it sounded pretty and it was the name I used to call my late grandfather, whom I adored.

The next day was more hectic than the streets of New Delhi. We had become parents overnight, but had not yet met or held our babies. I had previously informed my job I planned on finishing work and starting parental leave on the 4th of April, as it would give me a couple of days to get last minute packing done before we flew to India. However, some things cannot be planned and, in this case, I went into work that morning and excitedly announced at the manager's morning meeting my babies had come early and were born the night before. Everyone was delighted for us, but it meant I was going to need to finish up straight away. It really was no different than if I was pregnant and the babies came early, but still, I struggled with the thought of giving up work. I'd always had a job and, at the time, was the front office manager at a Perth hotel. I loved my job; I had a great team and wonderful managers.

Not going through the actual pregnancy when you got to feel the baby move, kick, and your body change made it difficult to one day have my life as I knew it and the next day become a mother. It just did not feel real. Even though my mind was frantic I had the biggest grin on my face.

The clinic emailed photos of Bane and Daya so we could see what our children looked like. They were both so tiny and were hooked up to machines to help them breathe for the first few days of their lives. Looking at the photos of the two most precious newborns was surreal. In one sense, I could not believe they were our babies but then looking at them made me think they were the babies we were always meant to have. I kept looking at the photos of them and telling them to hold on tight, as Mummy and Daddy would be there as soon as they could.

Our plan was to get the first flight we could out of Perth to New Delhi; due to a lack of communication on some required paperwork to be completed before departing it looked like we were going to have to delay our departure.

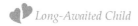

When we first sent our enquiry to our chosen clinic in New Delhi, we were also contacted by an Australian lady who was employed by the clinic to help assist with any questions we might have. She, along with another lady, had gone through the process of having their children with the same clinic in New Delhi and would be on hand right through the process to help us. Ian and I had no idea of the how, when, and whys of the process so we totally relied on the clinic and the two ladies in Australia to let us know what we had to do and when. I always said to them, "You tell me what I need to do and I will do it." Unfortunately, there had been a lack of communication and we were not advised that prior to leaving Australia to collect our babies Ian had to complete a DNA test sample. I was furious and beside myself, as it delayed our departure by five days. I kept chastising myself about being a mother who was not there when her babies were born and needed her. I know it was not our fault, but I was beating myself up over it.

I had followed all the steps as we were advised and still we had missed a crucial piece of information. When I questioned the staff about our misstep, their response was along the lines of we should have researched more or read blogs. That was not a good enough response in my opinion but all we could do was get the paperwork and tests done as quickly as possible. To be honest, once we had initially signed all the paperwork at the beginning of this journey I did not think there was much need for research as I thought we would be advised by our clinic of all we needed to know; thus, I did not follow any of the blogs from others on a similar journey. This was our journey and I did not want to read the highs of others in case we never reached that same point as parents, nor did I want to read about others losing their babies during pregnancy knowing it would be too upsetting for me. I just focused on us and what we needed to do.

My parents had visited a few weeks prior to the twins' unexpected early birth and my mum helped me shop for all the things we would need: blankets, clothing, bottles, formula, bibs, and more. As anyone who has prepared for a baby would know, there is a whole list of things you need to purchase for one baby, let alone two. Mum and I had a lot of fun doing this and looking through all the gorgeous baby outfits at the shops. Not to mention, Ian and I had bought two baby cots and a double stroller, ensuring it fit through the door of our apartment. I was now ready and prepared for this mummy job.

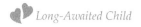

* * * *

When our babies were eight days old and I was already feeling like I was failing in the motherhood department for not being with them, we boarded our plane to New Delhi. What a difference nine months can make! The first time we had been waiting out in front of our apartment for our taxi to the airport, we had no idea what to expect in India and if it would even work for us. Nine months later we were again waiting for a taxi to the airport but were then giggly with all the excitement. We knew there was still a lot of paperwork to complete in India, but we had made it so far already and we would not let anything stop us.

For our flight to India, we booked Singapore Airlines, which was a lot more comfortable than our first flight to New Delhi. There would be no opening of the emergency exit door today! Our flight connection in Singapore meant we had a six-hour stopover at the airport so we booked a day pass to use the airport hotel pool. We could not wait to meet our babies and bring them back to Australia with us, but for ten years it had been just Ian and I—we were making sure we enjoyed every last minute of it just being the two of us.

Chapter 10

MEETING OUR
BABIES

The following day after we arrived late to New Delhi the night before, we took a taxi from our hotel to the hospital. This time around we decided to book the Fraser Suites, which was in the Mayur Vihar district of New Delhi. For us, when we looked on a map the distance to the hospital appeared about the same as our first hotel, the Imperial, only in a different direction.

The Fraser Suites was an apartment-style hotel with extra space plus a kitchen and laundry facilities that we thought would be handy to have. During our previous

95

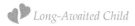

visit to New Delhi, we had a great driver who we ended up using the whole time we were there. He was polite and friendly, but most importantly, he knew the locations of the places we needed to go to, like the clinic and the hospital. I had kept his number for when we returned; on the morning we were to meet our babies for the first time, I gave the hotel receptionist the number of our driver, asking her to call him to see if he would collect us and take us to the hospital. She did not do as I had requested and booked another driver, whom she assured me knew where he was going. We assumed this was obviously a driver who provided the hotel a kickback. We had an appointment with the hospital to meet our newborn baby boy and baby girl for the first time at 9am; however, with the driver actually having no idea where he was going in the over populated city of New Delhi, we got lost numerous times. Two hours later we made it to the hospital. I was an emotional mess in the car. How could we be late to meet our babies for the first time? What would the nurses think of us?

Once inside, all the chaos was forgotten and the nursing staff did not even question us over our lack of punctuality. There we were standing at the door of the nursery ward looking through the glass windows at a row of babies sleeping peacefully in their cribs. There were two tiny newborns swaddled up and laying side by side in the same crib. Were they our babies? A lovely nurse handed us hospital gowns to wear over our clothes and we had to ensure our hands were washed with hospital grade sanitizer, just like we would if in Australia.

There Ian and I were about to meet our babies for the very first time. Our long-awaited moment finally came. The nurse took us to see the twins laying in the same crib. They were our babies! She handed me our son, Bane, and Ian was handed our daughter, Daya. *Wow! We were really parents!*

I could see Ian was totally in love with his little girl. We both were instantly in love with both of our children. We got to spend an hour with Bane and Daya, feeding and holding them and just staring at their beautiful little faces and perfect little hands. I had a few tears but in an extremely happy way. Then we were sent on our way and asked to bring back blankets, onesies, and nappies later that day. It was hard to leave but we planned on visiting them again that afternoon.

Apart from the warm clothing we had packed for them to wear home on the plane we had only packed light clothing for the babies, assuming they would not need full onesies in the very warm Indian climate. I was not aware newborn babies could not regulate their own temperature so they had to be fully dressed, even in 40-degree Celsius temperatures. We asked the nursing staff where a good place would be to shop and were informed the local Greater Kailash Markets had a variety of stores. We waved down a taxi outside the hospital and jumped in to head to the shops. Once again, outside each shop it was noisy and dirty but then once inside most of the stores it was no different to being in a store in Australia.

That afternoon we checked out of the Fraser Suites Hotel and back into the Imperial Hotel where we stayed on our first visit to New Delhi; it felt a lot safer and more like home to us. Plus, we were not going to risk being late to visit our babies again!

Over the next two days, we visited Bane and Daya a couple of times each day for feeding and changing. The nursing staff advised us we were not allowed to take our babies home with us immediately, instead we had to spend time with them in the hospital to allow the nurses time to know we were comfortable with feeding and changing the babies. After two days we were told if we came back that same afternoon we could take them home to the hotel with us. I do not in any way want anyone to think this was our first step in bad parenting; however, as I am being honest this is how Ian and I responded—we asked if we could return the following morning to pick them up instead. They said it was fine and they did not, thankfully, question us why. But, of course, they didn't; the nurses in the hospital were some of the most gorgeous and calm people I have ever met in my life. With our babies sleeping peacefully at the hospital Ian and I then went back to the hotel and spent the afternoon swimming in the gorgeous hotel pool, relaxing and enjoying a couple of cocktails. This really was the very last time it was going to be just us, so we made the most of it. It was a relaxing afternoon knowing we had pretty much come to the end of this journey. All we had to do was complete all paperwork efficiently and correctly and get back to Perth as soon as possible.

The following morning, we were at the hospital at 9am to take our babies home to the hotel with us. We could not get the silly grins off our faces, but we were just so proud—proud of ourselves for not letting anything stop us in our desire to be parents and already so proud of our babies for being so strong.

It was a strange feeling all of a sudden being parents without going through the pregnancy bit myself. It was like we had just been out shopping and purchased the most precious items ever. Even though we were included by email on Manu's pregnancy, we never got to see her growing bigger as she carried our babies. Most mothers-to-be have nine months to feel the baby growing inside them and going to prenatal classes for all the birthing tips and skills on being a first-time parent. Not us—we had to learn on the job.

On Monday, 25th March 2013, we left the hospital with our twin babies. We had them all snuggled up in their little Phil & Ted's cocoon carry bags. This was it—we were responsible for these two tiny human beings whom we loved with all our hearts. Back at the hotel, they became little celebrities amongst the staff as everywhere we went we were carrying them with us. This was the beginning of some of our most unbelievable moments—it was our life now.

We had been advised by the clinic to allow a minimum of three weeks in India to finalise all paperwork, which would allow the babies to come home to Australia with us. The staff at the clinic had sent us the name of a lady in New Delhi who assisted families going through the same process with all the paperwork and to help rush it through. That is what we wanted — to get all paperwork and formalities done and be back home in Perth with our babies. The woman charged $1000 for her services and it was most definitely worth it. Without her, we would not have really known where to start and in what order. We still had to do most of the running around to complete paperwork ourselves, but her guidance and knowledge were invaluable. She even asked us to have a couple of spare US$50 notes to slip in with the paperwork to get our applications put on the top of the pile at the offices.

Ian had to do another DNA test that would be sent back to Australia for confirmation along with the babies' DNA test samples. It was this formality that would take the longest time to be approved.

The babies also needed Australian citizenship, Australian emergency passports, and exit visas. Australian emergency passports are approved more rapidly than a normal passport and, at the time, were only valid for six months. Their passport photos were taken whilst they were still in the hospital. How the photographer got two newborn babies not even two weeks old to open their eyes for their passport photos I do not know. Their passports and photos are definitely keepers.

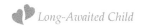

We had previously been informed that babies born through surrogacy agreements in India were born stateless, which meant they were not given Indian citizenship by virtue of the fact they were born in India. We had to apply for their Australian citizenship at the Australian consulate in India.

With regard to birth certificates, both parents' names appear on the birth certificate provided one parent has a genetic link with the child; therefore, Ian and I both have our names on their birth certificates even though I am not biologically the mother or the birth mother to Bane and Daya. The Delhi Municipal Council issued their birth certificates and advised to have our babies' birth certificates stamped with an apostille seal, an internationally recognised seal that gives the birth certificate legal validity in countries outside India.

Most days, we were out and about completing some form of paperwork or taking Bane and Daya to see the doctor for check-ups. They were very content newborn babies and would be happy to go along with us at any time, sleeping away in the cocoon bags. They were feeding well and the doctor was very happy with their weight gain. Day and night, Ian and I set an alarm for every three hours to remind us or wake us up to feed them 30ml of milk. They were always so sleepy and when giving them their bottles we would mimic the nurses from the hospital by quietly saying "Wake up, bayyybeee!" and rubbing their little noses or ears. Our hotel room was well set-up with a microwave for sterilising bottles and I hand washed all their little clothes in the bathroom sink and would have them hanging all around the room. The Indian weather was hot! Ian and I would want to have the air conditioner on all the time, however, as soon as we did, the babies did not like the cool air and would get upset. So, instead we had our first lesson as parents of putting your children first and kept the air-conditioner off, no matter how hot we were. We had our laptop with us and emailed photos and updates to our families back in Australia every day. They were all so excited to see the new little members of our family.

Whilst making the rounds of visiting offices, doctors, or the clinic, we would often run into other couples who were doing exactly the same thing as us. They had also recently met their newborn baby for the first time and were going through the steps to have their paperwork completed as soon as possible to get back to the country they were from. We would get talking and so many were envious of how we managed to have twins. For us, if we had one then we would be a one-child

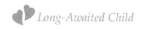

family, but most couples we met were adamant they would try surrogacy again, especially if they had frozen embryos.

After a week of being back at our hotel with our babies, I sent an email to the clinic asking if Manu would like to see the babies before she left the surrogate home where she had stayed with her family. The clinic replied saying Manu would like to see the babies, however, she did not wish to hold either of them, which we understood.

Before leaving Perth, I bought a gorgeous Swarovski gold bracelet with coloured stones throughout as a thank you gift for Manu along with extra Indian Rupee to the value of US$500 in a thank you card. I regret at the time not buying two bracelets so Daya could have had a matching one for herself, however at the time of purchasing this gift for Manu I was not aware we were even having a girl. I still go in to any Swarovski store I come across to check if they have one. I had asked the mum I met in the waiting room back at the clinic in New Delhi (on our first visit to India) what she had bought her surrogate and she said a saree, which was the most common gift. I, however, did not want to do this, as even though I saw so many gorgeous sarees, I was unsure what was classed as fashionable. I was happy with my gift for Manu and hoped the extra money helped her and her family and the bracelet may help her feel a little closer to and remember the babies she once carried.

The next day, we went to the clinic for our appointment with Manu. Ian and I were waiting in a room for her along with Bane and Daya. The moment Manu walked in I will never forget and I never want to, as it is a constant reminder of this selfless, amazing woman and what she did for us. Manu instantly broke down in tears upon seeing the babies in our arms. It was the type of emotion that has you doubled over with heartache. I hugged her and I cried along with her. After a couple of minutes, Manu managed to control herself, however I was a blubbering mess the whole time. My mind kept putting me in her shoes; she had carried these babies for 33 weeks and been able to listen to their heartbeats and feel them move inside her body. Even though they were not hers biologically, they were a part of her. I cannot imagine the heartache knowing she would most likely never see them again.

Manu could not speak English so we had an interpreter in the room. We hugged Manu and told her we could never thank her enough. This one moment, saying goodbye to Manu, broke my heart into a million pieces, more so than any negative pregnancy test result. There is not a day that goes by that I do not think of Manu and how grateful I am for the part she played in making our dream of being a family come true. I would do anything to be able to see her again and give her a big hug. I hope she has moved on from the loss she would have felt, and has instead focused on the opportunities the money has been able to provide her and her family.

Some days we had to sit and wait for the call that some paperwork was ready to be collected. On these days we would sit in the cool by the hotel pool with our babies or on one particular day we all went to a local market. I bought some beautiful keepsake pieces for our twins. Besides the gorgeous cot blankets with Indian elephants on them, I bought Bane an Indian antique blue brass vase and Daya a gorgeous pink mosaic and silver bowl. These are pieces I hope they will cherish as they get older. I also bought gorgeous pink and blue photo albums with the intent to put photos, emails and stories of how they came about.

It took 21 days for our paperwork to be finalised. On our last day in New Delhi, our final pieces of paperwork, the exit visas for Bane and Daya, were completed. The completion involved the four of us going to an office, essentially a partially outside room with no air-conditioning, to get the exit visas approved. After sitting in the extreme heat for three hours waiting for our number to be called, I asked one of the staff members if it would be all right for Ian to take the babies back to the hotel, as it was not a healthy environment for the babies to be in let alone feed in, and I would stay behind to finalise the paperwork. Thankfully, this was allowed. Ian may be the researcher but I was the one who handled these trying situations better. I sat in that room from 9am to 5pm. During one stage of the interview, I was questioned on my marriage with Ian. Due to the recent change of law, we had been informed by the clinic to act like we were married. I explained we were married, however, I had kept my maiden name as it was on my passport. Thankfully, I had a ring on my wedding finger, which Ian had bought for me some years ago, and I showed it to the officer; he trusted what I said and stamped the exit visas giving us permission to take Bane and Daya out of the country. I am not sure what would have happened if I had said we were not married!

Finally, at 5.30 pm, after our driver collected me, I made it back to the hotel. We were free to leave the country the following morning. It was all such

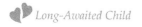

an overwhelming process that we never thought we could relax and feel safe until we were back home in Australia.

After sitting in that room all day, in the heat feeling very anxious, I needed a shower, a cuddle with my babies followed by a lovely, family dinner in the hotel restaurant to celebrate.

Chapter 11

HOMEWARD BOUND

Our final goodbye to the Imperial Hotel and the amazing staff who worked there was on 10th April 2013. We think we will take Bane and Daya back to New Delhi one day when they are older and, of course, we will stay at the beautiful Imperial Hotel. It is, after all, the home address on their birth certificates! Amongst all the chaos of New Delhi, it is a beautiful and vibrant city and it had been our first home with our babies. I had mixed emotions on our way to the airport. We had been in India for three weeks so I was excited to be finally going home as

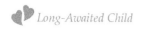

a family of four, but also sad to be saying goodbye to the country where my babies were born and their surrogate mother lived.

Just before we had left New Delhi, Bane started to appear distressed and uncomfortable when having his bottle. My mother's intuition must have clicked in, as without much knowledge on the subject my mind immediately knew it was colic. Some mums and doctors believe there is such a thing, some do not. After seeing Bane cry and being so uncomfortable, I did. I Googled all sorts of remedies with only one option of some medicine available at a chemist in New Delhi. In the middle of the night, I sent Ian off in a taxi to a chemist that was open to get whatever he could find. The medicine seemed to ease the pain for Bane a little for the time being. It was frustrating researching knowing there would be more options to help my son when we returned to Australia. We just had to get there.

Once again, Singapore Airlines was amazing for our return flight. The staff took great care of us and our precious little cargo. They were so attentive helping us board and assisting us during our flight. We were now one of those couples who got to board first because we had young children! Love that perk, as with two tiny babies it gave us time to settle in before take-off.

We had booked two seats with two bassinets. Due to one bassinet taking up the space in front of two seats, the airline had given us four seats in the middle section of the plane with two bassinets along the wall in front of us. It was perfect as it gave us so much more room to spread out and made the whole flight more bearable. Having to give bottles every few hours along with nappy changes in the toilets, you can imagine the amount of carry-on luggage we had on the plane. The airline crew fussed over these two little babies and I am sure everyone could see Ian and I beaming with pride.

We had decided to stop overnight in Singapore, staying at the Rendezvous Hotel again, to give the babies, and us, a rest from the six-hour flight. Looking back now, I am impressed by how Ian and I just took our new parenting roles in stride. We had no classes beforehand to tell us how the parenting business worked nor had we read any books, though maybe I should have; however, we just learnt as we went along and I think we did pretty well.

Before we flew out of Singapore the following morning for our final flight back to Perth I got the chance to do a little shopping—not for me though. This time it was all about my babies at Baby Gap.

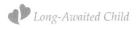

When checking in at the International Airport at Singapore, a lady checking in at the counter next to us looked over at us and noticed our babies sleeping in their cocoons. This was the conversation I had with her:

Lady: "Do you have babies in there?"

Me: "Yes, they are only three weeks old."

Lady: "Have you just had twins?"

Me: "Yes."

Lady: "Oh my God, you look amazing."

Me: "Why, thank you."

I never explained to her how I never actually carried my babies myself; I just enjoyed this little moment of feeling like a celebrity who loses all her baby weight within five minutes of giving birth. It still gives me a little smile when I think of it.

Landing at Perth Airport and getting through customs without any issues was the biggest relief. It was a cold night in Perth compared to the humidity of India, but it did not matter, nor did the fact it was midnight when our flight landed, as we were happy to be home in our own country. Ian later told me he feared the plane was going to be instructed to divert back to India with some scary-looking authority boarding the plane and taking our babies from us. This could not happen as the babies were biologically his, but we truly never believed everything was going to be okay until we had our babies back in Australia with us. It had been a long process and words cannot describe how relieved, albeit exhausted, we were.

We stood in the long taxi queue patiently waiting our turn. Our babies were rugged up inside their little cocoons; so as long as they were happy, we were not going to let the cold or the long line up make this moment anything but completely joyous.

It was about 1am when we arrived back at our apartment. Three weeks earlier it had been just Ian and I waiting out front for our taxi to the airport and now there we were arriving back home with our twin babies. Our journey to have a family of our own was now complete.

That night back in our apartment, giving Bane and Daya their bottles and settling them into their cots was a moment of sheer happiness. I didn't sleep much that night, as I was constantly checking on them and seeing if this had all really happened and it was not just a dream. Luckily, for Ian and me, our dreams had finally come true.

Chapter 12

BACK HOME IN PERTH

In the morning after we arrived home, we phoned our families to let them know we were home safe. Everyone was so excited and also a little relieved that we made it back without any issues. It was planned that Ian's family would be first to visit followed by mine. Everyone who knew about the gorgeous little additions to our family were busting to meet them.

There were still many people in our lives who had no idea we had even become parents. This may sound strange and unfair to have not said anything, but I

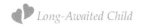

truly did not believe we were going to become parents and everything would be all right until the four of us were safely back in our apartment in Perth.

A short time after arriving home, I posted a message on Facebook along with a photo of our gorgeous twins: "Our baby twin boy & girl born 13th March — Bane Max Nielsen & Daya Poppy Nielsen." Most of the comments received back were positive, with friends so excited for us; however, there were a few comments and messages where I could read between the lines that some were shocked we hadn't told them we were even pregnant beforehand. It may sound unfounded, but to me it wasn't about them; if only some of these friends knew what we had been through and the obstacles we hurdled to get to the point of actually having our babies, then maybe they would understand why we kept this so close to our chests. But, I never told them of our struggles, so their feelings of being left out was not entirely misunderstood. I had to let go of any negativity though, as I had bigger things to worry about now in the form of two little human beings.

We have friends and family who know the babies were born in India by surrogate, yet we have never really told everyone we used an egg donor. It was all on a need-to-know basis and as far as Ian and I were concerned, Bane and Daya were our babies and that was all anyone needed to know. They both have features and make facial expressions like Ian so I am sure people can figure out they are not biologically mine due to Bane and Daya's dark features. But I love the ones who have not mentioned or cared about this and love Bane and Daya for who they are, our gorgeous little babies.

For a long time after returning home I still had my insecurities over others' opinions. I had to repeatedly tell myself they were our babies and how they were conceived or brought into this world was really no one else's business. I have never heard anyone question another person who, for example, may have adopted a child or ask a mother if her baby was actually hers, so it truly amazed me how brazen strangers and friends were to ask such a question. If they asked if they were mine, I would reply "Of course they are," with an expression that said "How could you even ask such a stupid question?" Like I said, it did not matter how my children were brought into this world; I was (am) their mother and Ian their father. I have had to, at times, walk away from friendships due to the questions and negativity I received. Some of these friends I have connected with again, however there are some friendships

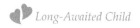

that sadly will never be the same. When you think about it, it is very sad that friendships can fall apart over Ian and I just trying every possible angle to have a family and wanting to keep some of the details private.

In saying all that, we have some amazing family and friends in our lives. Some know the whole truth and some don't (but it obviously does not matter to them), but all have doted on our children and have been amazing support for Ian and me.

My mum came over to visit us in Perth often and was there for my first Mother's Day. She, Bane, Daya, and I all went out to celebrate and enjoy a lovely high tea in a beautiful winery in Swan Valley, north of Perth City. That was a really special day to share with my Mum and one I waited almost a decade to experience.

For the first six months after arriving back in Perth, I had to take Bane and Daya to a paediatrician every fortnight for check-ups. Our paediatrician was a lovely old lady, albeit a very honest and at times brutal one. She had been a doctor specialising in paediatrics for over 50 years and was the old-fashioned type of doctor who told you as it was and did not believe in babies developing colic.

One visit I was trying to explain to her the pain Bane

appeared to be in at night and when I mentioned colic she responded with "Rubbish!" I told her how it was more comfortable for Bane to be on his stomach, and as I was always worried about having him lying on his stomach in his cot, instead I would have him lying on his stomach on my chest as I lay on the couch. She did not agree and snapped saying, "Do you want your baby to die?" I burst into tears. Of course, I did not want my baby to die! I thought I had been doing the right thing so this way I could always hear him breathing. It made me feel terrible. I loved my babies, I loved being a Mummy and with Ian working away I was trying to do the best I could with most of the time being on my own.

She was a very caring, thorough doctor though. During one visit, she had me rush Bane to the hospital across the road to have some tests done without even explaining what the tests were for. Thankfully, my mum was visiting again so she looked after Daya. Once I arrived at the hospital, the nurses took Bane away from me for tests though I still did not know what was going on. Our paediatrician came to the hospital once the testing was done to let me know all was okay; she had been concerned he had a heart condition. My poor boy had already been through so much! Still now I worry about him.

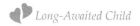

It was a good thing the doctor did have x-rays done on Bane's chest as it did show his rib cage was thin and not developing as it should, which would most likely be due to a Vitamin D deficiency. This is a common condition with a large part of Indian population due to their dark skin, as the pigment melanin can reduce the skin's ability to produce Vitamin D from the sun. It is however more common in women than in men because of certain social and cultural customs that dictate lifestyle patterns such as clothing and diet. Both Bane and Daya had blood tests to check and they were both highly deficient, therefore I was given medication for them to take for the next six months. I am so thankful the doctor picked this up, otherwise we may have had some issues down the track as too little Vitamin D in children can result in soft or fragile bones.

Apart from that, they were both happy babies and continued to develop and grow in the normal chart range. After six months it was just monthly visits until their first birthday. Bane's tummy pains and colic was a struggle for the first six months of his little life. It took a few attempts to get the right formula and type of bottle for him to feed from where he did not take in gulps of air along with the milk, allowing him to feel better and not endure so much pain. I didn't have a mother's group to confide in or ask questions. I just researched and read reviews that Dr Brown's bottles were the best for colic and I agreed, and I ended up switching to these bottles for both Bane and Daya, just as a cautionary act. Also, searching for remedies on the Internet I came across a medicine formulated in Victoria, which made all the difference. This stuff was worth its weight in gold. Unfortunately, it was a little hard to get your hands on at times due to the word getting around and it selling out quickly.

Unfortunately, our move to Perth a few years earlier meant we did not have family close by to help with Bane and Daya; however, family and friends often visited from the East Coast who wanted to meet the twins for the first time. It was a big help having them there with me with Ian working away. On a few occasions two of my girlfriends from the east coast visited. Boy, were these completely different visits to any prior to the twins being born! Now it was walks along the river, visits to parks and lunches out, compared to shopping and afternoon drinks at a trendy bar, but they did not mind. With not having children of their own, they absolutely adored and spoilt Bane and Daya, and still do to this day.

I did have an older wonderful staff member who

had worked for me at the Perth Hotel, who had also became a close friend and helped me with Bane and Daya. Oh, how I needed her assistance! She was like another grandma to my babies and would come along to many outings with us from nursery rhyme time at the local library to the doctors for their vaccinations. Occasionally I would drop them over to her place for a couple of hours, telling her I was going home to catch up on the housework but would end up walking in the door of my apartment and falling asleep on the bed. At times, I was exhausted. Just for me to go out in the car I had to put them both in the double stroller, take them down the lift to the apartment carpark, put them in the car, fold the stroller up, put it in the boot, and then do the reverse when we got home.

Of course, it was always the most fun when Ian came home. He missed a lot since he worked away from home, but he was a good provider for his family. The costs involved to have our family put us behind, although we would not change it for the world. I was constantly taking photos and videos of our twins to send to him.

During the times I was on my own with the babies, I had to often think outside the box. Two examples that come to mind are when they had grown out of their baby bath, and then outgrown the laundry tub; without a bath in our apartment I had to bathe them in the shower. It was difficult to do so I bought an Ikea plastic highchair without the tray for each to sit in when having their shower. They loved it. The next trick was for car excursions, since Daya would scream like a banshee if she could not see me (as at the time she was rear-facing). Though I had a toy mirror sitting on the back seat, it did not help. So, I took a happy photo of myself, had it blown up to A4 size, and stuck it on the back seat. She was happy she could see Mummy all the time! I look forward to telling them stories like these when they are older.

The following November I turned 40. I didn't need a party as all I wanted was to go away with my little family of four to my favourite spot in Western Australia, the Pullman Hotel in Bunker Bay. In my 20s, I had imagined I would become a mum in my early 30s (without a thought that I would have fertility issues). As time went by, my mummy deadline increased from 34 to 36 to 38. When I didn't think it was going to happen by the time I turned 40, this age deadline changed to 42, however none of that mattered now as there I was on my 40th birthday with my two gorgeous babies and supportive partner in

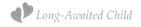

a gorgeous part of the country feeling like I did not want or need anything else in my life.

Just after the twins' first birthday in March 2014, we made the decision to move back to Queensland. Considering both of our parents lived in Queensland, we wanted Bane and Daya to grow up knowing and having a lovely relationship with their grandparents. They had all been such a big support for us; we knew they deserved the right to also have the twins as a big part of their lives as well.

We packed up our belongings and shipped everything home. We said our very sad goodbyes to our friends — some of whom will always have a special place in my heart — my work colleagues and our apartment. Then, we bundled the four of us up, along with the supplies we needed, for a four-week drive back across the Nullarbor Plain via Tasmania. With two 12-month old children, were we crazy to take such a journey? Nevertheless, as Ian and I were used to doing, we took everything in our stride and, somehow, we all survived. We even caught the ferry over to Tasmania to visit my grandmother, Nanna, in Hobart so she could meet her great-grandchildren for the first time. I am so grateful we did this as Nanna passed away a few months later.

Overall, it was an interesting four-week drive from Perth to Queensland. A couple of stages along the way the babies were sick, which ended in a few hospital visits. We stopped at Canberra for a couple of nights as Ian and I had always wanted to go to the War Memorial. Unfortunately, we were only there for five minutes when Bane projectile vomited on the carpet. I felt terrible as it was such a sacred and heart-warming place and there was my son throwing up on the floor at the Anzac display. We cleaned it up, apologised over and over, and headed back to the hospital once again.

This hospital visit they finally tested him and, as it turned out, he had salmonella poisoning. Though we were unsure how he got it, it was another moment of feeling like I was failing as a mummy. My boy was so sick and it broke my heart. It took a long seven days for him to be well again and go back to the happy little boy we loved so much.

On top of that drama, the straps holding the double pram on the roof rack came loose, which sent it flying off onto the (thankfully) deserted part of the highway. Not to mention, we also had the twin's porta-cots stolen from the roof of the car in the hotel carpark in Newcastle. Apart from those few productions, we made a load of wonderful memories and it certainly

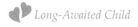

was a trip to remember. I hope one day to take the kids on a 12-month caravan trip doing a full lap exploring our wonderful country. I am sure there will be more drama then as well, but also the chance to build so many memories to cherish.

Once back in Queensland, we decided to stay in Hervey Bay for a while and live with my parents. They were a big help as I also returned to work. When the twins were 18-months old, Ian and I went on an overseas holiday with my sister and a few friends to America to celebrate our 40th birthdays, although at almost 41, I was the oldest in my group of friends. It was the first time we had left Bane and Daya, but they were going to be spending time with my parents and aunty who had come up from Tasmania to help out. It was a fun holiday but to be away from Bane and Daya for a couple of weeks was really hard at times. I missed them like crazy.

Not long after we got home from our holiday, I was not feeling my best and had become extremely emotional. I kept brushing it all aside thinking I was just a tired, working mum of twin toddlers. One morning, when Ian was driving me to work, I told him to take me to the hospital instead. I was a complete mess emotionally and had started bleeding. The doctor asked if I could possibly be pregnant, which I responded to with a very certain "No way!" I gave her a brief rundown on my fertility struggles and our babies being surrogate babies and that it could possibly be that cysts had formed on my uterus again. The doctor did a blood test and the next day I was to return for the results. That night, I lay in bed wondering, if I was pregnant would I actually want another baby? Yes, this baby would be Ian's and my biological child together, but I was now 41 and already tired from two little ones. I felt terrible for even considering I would not want this baby. I knew deep down if I were pregnant, it may take a little time to get used to the idea, but it would be so exciting.

So, the next morning I returned to the hospital for my results. Life really can feel terribly cruel at times, as after all I had been through, I had in fact been pregnant and the bleeding was caused by me miscarrying. Maybe it was the relaxed holiday vibe mixed with some cocktails that helped my body finally decide to relax and fall pregnant. I would not know, but once again it seemed my body did not actually want to carry a baby. Turns out, it was the hormones going nuts in my body from the miscarriage that had caused the emotions. I allowed myself to grieve the baby I would never carry or feel growing inside my body, but then I just had to

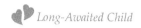

let it go. After all, I had my ultimate dream of having a family with Ian, Bane, and Daya.

Chapter 13

FIVE YEARS ON

Five years later and life is really good. When Bane and Daya were two, we moved back to the Sunshine Coast. We have built our forever family home and made some lovely friends through the school Bane and Daya attend.

Bane and Daya have grown into beautiful children with big hearts. Time is going by so quickly. It feels like it has all gone by in one big, fun blur. To be honest, I can hardly remember them being little babies. We often look at photos together and are amazed by how little they once were.

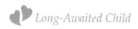

When Bane and Daya started talking and could say the words Mummy and Daddy, it took Ian and me a long time to stop becoming giddy at this. Still now, we occasionally look at each other and smile when we hear those precious words come from our children's beautiful little voices.

Every year just after Bane and Daya's birthday I send an email to our surrogacy clinic in New Delhi with photos of the twins, asking the staff to forward the pictures to Manu. I truly hope they do make it to her. I think of Manu every day when my children wake up and I see their faces; they are like gifts I receive over and over again. I wonder if Manu thinks of the two little babies she carried and gave birth to back in March 2013. For all I know, she may have been a surrogate again for another family, but wherever she is I hope she is happy and at peace.

Looking back, if I could change things so Ian and I could have our babies naturally I do not think I would. I love our story, as it brought out the strength and persistence in both of us. I am so proud of us for not letting ourselves be beaten down even on the days when we thought we had been. We have two amazing children who bring so much joy to our lives with every breath they take.

Bane is our little softy with the sweetest nature. He loves life and everyone in it, which is evident by the constant smile on his face. I love this about him. Daya is our little entertainer who gives most things a go. She is very funny but at the same time can be extremely emotional. They have a lovely, close relationship and it is a real joy to hear them laughing and playing together. I hope this never changes.

My wish for Bane and Daya growing up is for them is to continue to be the kind, caring people they already are, and to know how much they are loved and how much they were wanted. When kissing them goodnight, I often tell them I am so lucky to have them as my babies. Deep down I could not imagine having any other babies, even if it meant they were biologically mine.

Both Bane and Daya have features like Ian. I occasionally look at Daya, especially, and think how she looks nothing like me. I see other mums with their children who look so much like them and at times this rips at my heartstrings. Daya is starting to ask questions, like why she has brown eyes but I have blue. Ian and I have not gone down the path of how they were born yet, as we feel they are too young for this, but we have started to mention small things, like being born in

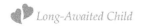

India. We will have these discussions with them when we feel the time is right.

Bane is the most carefree, happy-natured person so when the time comes for us to sit down and tell them the whole story, I do not think there will be any concern for him. Daya can be tempestuous and, while we have such a lovely, strong mother-daughter bond, I worry there will be repercussions. I fear one day when she is in her difficult teenage years and not getting her way she will yell at me, "You are not my real mother!" I know she will not mean it, but the thought breaks my heart.

After five years, I am not as insecure about my story. Up until now, I have not felt the need to tell just anyone; however, if something comes up in conversation with people I feel comfortable around I no longer feel embarrassed to say my children were born by surrogacy. Mostly, the situation arises around other mothers who seem to have an understanding of what it takes to be a mother and, possibly, they had their own struggles in the past. One thing I have learnt is to never ask, "When are you having children?" or anything of a similar nature. You just never know what anyone is going through behind closed doors.

The same can be said about Mother's Day. I like to take some time on that day to reflect on how fortunate I am to have two wonderful children in my life showering me with love. However, I will never forget the struggles we went through and how anyone out there could possibly be going through their own struggles. Before my children came into my world, Mother's Day depressed me, so I am very aware of how other people could be feeling on that particular day. For this reason, I never post on any social media about my Mother's Day.

I know there may be people who will have opinions on my story and not agree with surrogacy. Everyone seems to have an opinion these days. Not long ago, I saw a post on Facebook about a gay couple from the USA bringing home a baby after using a surrogate mother; it was a lovely story and these two men obviously longed to be parents and were so ecstatic with their dream coming true. Still, a person, a total stranger to these men, felt compelled to put her opinion forward. She did not agree with surrogacy and believed the baby would forever have an eternal sadness inside and long for the birth mother. I know she is entitled to her opinion, as we all are, however, until you have walked in someone else's shoes, I personally think we could all be a little more gentle with our opinions. I am fairly positive when it comes time to tell Bane and Daya about how they came into the world they will have a lot of questions. At the end of the day, if we had not used a surrogate mother and egg donor, my children would not exist; and you cannot find two children who are loved more.

As I have got older (and obviously wiser), I have started to believe in the notion that what you put out to the universe will come back to you. When Ian and I first moved in together, way back before we thought about trying for a baby, I bought two gorgeous Asian twin baby statues that I had fallen in love with for our garden. Fast forward fifteen years and it makes me wonder when I look at the statues in the garden if, at the time I purchased them, without realising or knowing I was going to need help, I put that sign out into the universe.

When mentioning this book to friends I am often asked how long it took me to finish writing. Most people are quite surprised when I say approximately seven months, as they believe this is not really a long time; however, I have had this book inside me for five years now, wanting to come out since our surrogate became pregnant. It really is quite ironic I have written a book, as I have hardly read a book of my own choosing since my babies were born five years ago.

Being the mother of twins has taken up my time and the years are going by so fast, but it felt like the right time and I hope my story will connect with anyone going through, or possibly about to start, a similar journey. If this is you, please understand you are not alone. While there are no guarantees, I hope reading my story makes yours a whole lot easier knowing someone else has been there.

My advice would be that if you really, truly want to be a parent, whether you are in a relationship or not, look into every possible option. I cannot imagine my life without Bane and Daya and sometimes wonder what I would be doing if Ian and I had not looked into surrogacy. Yes, it is very hard financially at times; overall, we spent well over $140,000 to be a family. That is a lot of money that could have been used to pay off a mortgage or to travel the world with, but for us, it has been the most rewarding money ever spent. So, work out how much you are prepared to spend and how much time you have to give and then go for it. Also, remember it is *your* journey—how you decide to deal with each situation and whom you decide to talk to is totally your own decision. Plus remember to be

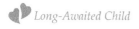

kind to yourself. It is not an easy journey, but you are already amazing for coming this far.

Apart from having our babies, writing this book has been one of my greatest achievements. I believe our baby journey and me writing this book is my path in life and I am so happy I have been able to share my journey with you. I wish anyone going through fertility struggles lots of love and pray you will also have your long-awaited moment. And for those who have children—I am sure you already do this—hold them tight and treasure every moment.

AFTERWORD

Kellie is my second child. She has always been kind-hearted and caring. I knew she would make a great mum one day.

Kellie's older sister, Jodie, was the first of our children to have a baby. Kellie still lived at home when our little granddaughter, and Kellie's niece, Emma, was born. Kellie adored Emma. She would drive over to her sister's place on a Saturday morning, bundle Emma up, and take her out for the day to visit her friends, giving Jodie some much needed time to rest or do housework. Kellie was so proud of her little niece and loved showing her off. Even though Emma is now in her 20s, Kellie

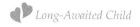

and Emma still have a beautiful relationship to this day.

For Kellie at the time, she must have just innocently assumed that when she met the right man she would settle down and have babies of her own. I remember when Kellie was about 18 years old and the little boy next door would crawl through a hole in the fence we had made for him. He loved coming over to have breakfast with Kellie or to play games. She was so patient and caring towards him. Even though many years have passed, it makes us laugh knowing the connection this 18-year-old girl had with the little two-year-old boy next door. We have many lovely memories of those times and we are still close with the family from next door.

Kellie adores her nieces and nephews and even though she eventually left home, it did not matter where in Australia or overseas she was living as she always took the time to ring and keep in contact.

When Kellie and Ian met and the time was right, they wanted to start a family of their own. At the time, no one could have predicted that simple, natural decision would take them on such a rollercoaster of a ride.

One day Kellie came to me and told me they were going to start IVF treatment. She explained they had been trying to conceive naturally for a long time but were unable to, even though the tests they had showed everything was fine. It was agonising seeing her injecting the IVF hormones into her body; her stomach was bruised, she was emotional, and her moods were up and down. It was hard to see someone I loved so much suffering. There was nothing I could do but be there for her when she needed or wanted me to—that was a difficult thing for me, being her mother.

During one of her IVF cycles, I went along with Kellie for the embryo transfer and, up until that point, everything had gone accordingly and we were all feeling extremely positive that this time it was going to work. However, on arrival at the clinic the doctor told us the embryos were not developing and if they did the transfer they would most likely not implant, as they were just not healthy enough. Kellie was devastated and this was the first time I saw for myself what she had to go through emotionally. I tried pulling myself together to be brave for her, as I didn't want Kellie to see my tears, but my heart was breaking for her. As her mother, and knowing everything she had gone through, to be told it wasn't going to work this time was crippling. I could see it was even difficult for the staff at the clinic to fight back their own tears. The

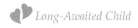

doctor decided to do the transfer procedure anyway; however, I knew in my heart it was only because we could all see Kellie was clinging onto any chance of hope it may work.

Unfortunately, for Kellie and Ian this was another negative pregnancy test. They were distraught. I honestly thought it would be the last time they tried, as the disappointments had really started to take their toll on them both emotionally and financially, but again Kellie's continued strength and determination proved me wrong.

Six months later, Kellie and Ian decided to try a clinic in Brisbane. I felt this was definitely going to be their last attempt as Kellie was not well after the egg retrieval surgery. I went down to stay with them and help Kellie during the day. I saw the look in Ian's eyes—he was very concerned for Kellie and the impact it had on her mind and body. Once again, it was a negative result. We cried for Ian and Kellie.

As Kellie's mother, my heart was aching and I spent many nights lying awake worrying about her and whether it was all worth it. It was made harder by the fact I could not do anything for her apart from being there when she needed me to be, listen to her decisions, and encourage her through them, even when there was no certainty in any of them.

Eventually it all became too much for them and they decided to take a break from it all and moved to Perth. This would be a chance for Ian to start a new job and for them to catch up financially, as the cost of continuous IVF cycles certainly put a strain on their finances.

After being in Perth for some time, Kellie rang me and said they were going to try IVF one more time. I would listen to her and could sense her grasping onto hope that this time it might happen. Unfortunately, this was another negative pregnancy result for them. When Kellie rang to tell me the news, all I could do was cry. It was just not fair; there are so many children in unloving homes and here were two people who would make wonderful parents having to put themselves through so much to have a family.

In 2012, my husband, Max, and I were on a cruise; we had one stop in Jerusalem. We went on a tour to Old Jerusalem, where Jesus walked with the cross and then onto the Wailing Wall. I spoke to a lady I had met and told her the heartbreak Kellie and Ian were going through and I was going to put a note of prayer in the Wailing Wall for them. .After returning to the bus, that

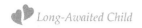

same lady came to tell me she also put a note in the wall for Kellie. I was very moved by her lovely gesture and that a complete stranger could be so kind.

When we returned home, Kellie and Ian told us they had looked into surrogacy in India rather than try IVF again. At first, we were nervous as we did not know anything about surrogacy or that international surrogacy could be an option. They explained to us how it all worked and even though we still had our doubts, we were also hopeful. Before we knew it, they were off to India. There was really no stopping those two.

They returned to Australia very happy with how everything went; not long after, Kellie rang excitedly with the news they had received an email from the clinic in India to say their surrogate mother was pregnant. They were over the moon and we were so elated for them, we could not sleep. We did not know at the time we were actually going to get two gorgeous grandchildren.

Later that year, we were caravanning in Western Australia on our way down to Perth to spend Christmas with Kellie and Ian. Jodie, Kellie's sister, and her family also came across for our family Christmas. Kellie and Ian were so excited about having twins and they could not believe their dream was coming true. We had a beautiful Christmas that year with all the family making plans to visit when the twins came home to Australia.

After Christmas, we continued on our way in the caravan. It was late one night when we received a call from Kellie—their twin babies had been born! We had a new little grandson and granddaughter. Kellie and Ian's dream had finally come true in what was their last attempt to have a family of their own. We were all overcome with joy and tears began to flow. They not only had their own baby, they had two, and an instant family—a brother and a sister for each other.

Kellie and Ian flew to India as soon as they could to meet their new little babies and bring them home to Australia. Kellie sent photos every day. One photo in particular I will always remember was of Ian holding Daya; she was not much bigger than his hand. Kellie just kept saying over and over how beautiful they were. We were so thrilled she and Ian were finally a mum and a dad. Max was so proud when they chose his name for Bane's middle name; I knew it meant the world to him.

Once they had all the paperwork and Australian

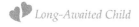*Long-Awaited Child*

passports arranged they flew home with their two tiny babies. When they arrived back home in Perth, Ian had some time at home with Kellie and the babies but he did have to go back to work. I arranged to fly over to see my beautiful grandchildren and to help Kellie in whatever way I could. I could not wait! So far, I had only seen photos.

When I arrived at the apartment, Kellie looked exhausted so I got her to write down the feeding routine and sent her straight to bed. Between the two of us, we soon had a good system of writing down feeding times as the babies needed to be fed every three hours. I loved my time with Kellie, Bane, and Daya. They had an apartment in Perth city, so we often went for walks along the river or to the shops. It was fun shopping for the babies. We even had our favourite lunch spot at the David Jones Café where we could easily manoeuvre the double pram to a table. My time there was so special and what made it even more so was spending Kellie's first Mother's Day with her and her babies.

I was very sad and teary as I had to return home to Hervey Bay but Kellie decided they would fly back with me so the whole family could meet Bane and Daya. After a couple of weeks, they returned to Perth with Kellie's lovely friend Peita flying back with her.

144

Two babies meant there needed to be two adults travelling to nurse them. Ian was at home one out of five weeks and he was fantastic helping Kellie and giving her time to catch up on sleep. Kellie had the occasional friend and family member visiting, but apart from that, she did an amazing job coping with twins.

Not long after Daya and Bane turned one, Kellie and Ian decided to move back to Hervey Bay. They packed up the car to make the long drive home via Tasmania to visit Kellie's nanna and aunty who lived in Hobart. Max and I flew down as well and we all had a wonderful time together. It was lovely to see my mother meeting her new great grandchildren before sadly passing away three months later.

Once back in Hervey Bay, Kellie and her family came to live with us for a while. Ian still worked interstate and came back for his week off. Kellie found some part-time work and put Daya and Bane into daycare a couple of days a week. Max and I would walk up to the daycare centre in the afternoon to pick them up; it was always a delight seeing their little excited faces. We grew so close and loved this special time with them. When walking home with the twins in their strollers, Daya would look over her shoulder at her Pa and Bane would chatter or sing the whole way home. I

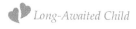

often looked at them and thought "Our little miracles." We have such wonderful memories to treasure. They all finally moved back to their home on the Sunshine Coast. It is only a couple of hours away but we miss seeing their smiling faces every day.

It took Kellie and Ian eight long, agonising, and emotional years to have a family, but no matter how hard the going got, Kellie never gave up on the hope of being a mum. It truly has been a miracle. Bane and Daya have made those gruelling years so worthwhile and we could not image our life without them.

I hope anyone reading Kellie's story that may be having similar struggles will be inspired by what Kellie and Ian have achieved. Through all the ups and downs, the pain and the heartache, dreams can come true and miracles really can happen. I hope for a miracle for you.

With love,
Pauline Harriden
Kellie's Mum, Bane and Daya's Granny

THANK YOU

To Ian: Thank you for your patience, sense of humour, and love of researching the big decisions in our life. This is OUR story, which I would not have any other way. I cannot imagine going on this journey with anyone else but you, and I know it was just as difficult and emotional at times for you as it was for me. Thank you for being so strong for both of us.

To my parents, Max and Pauline Harriden: I cannot thank you enough for all your support. I know at times how hard it was for you both to see us going through this but we got there in the end. Thank you for being the best Granny and Pa my children could

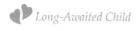

ask for. We all love you so much.

To my sister Jodie: Thank you for having your three gorgeous children. You know I loved each of them as if they were my own from the moment they were born. You having your children and seeing how beautiful your relationship with them is made me want to be a mother myself.

To my gorgeous girlfriends: Thank you. I truly hope you all know who you are. I am so lucky to have so many of you spread over our wonderful country and even overseas. So many of you have been such a support for me at some stage during this journey and still continue to be such a big part of Bane and Daya's lives. Thank you to those who have only recently come into my life and have been my cheer squad for me completing this book. I love you all and cannot wait to celebrate with you.

To my wonderful friend, Peita: I cannot do my thank you without mentioning you. You were the leader of my tribe. From day one of saying we were doing IVF right up until we had Bane and Daya, you were the friend I needed. Our drive home from work chats where we solved all the problems of the world were at times my lifesaver. You listened to my craziness, my tears, and my joy without any hesitation but to keep listening. You really are a good egg.

To my mentor, Rachael Bermingham: Thank you for your guidance, honesty, and sharing your knowledge, which has been invaluable to me. You have kept me accountable to my commitment to write my story, a dream of mine for five years. It was not until I met you at one of your workshops that I knew my dream could really come true. It has taken me many months of tapping away at my computer (and at times many tears) reliving my journey, but it has all been so worth it. I am so thankful you came into my life. Plus, thank you to your team at Bermingham Books for their patience and helping me put it all together at the end.

Ian and I feel very lucky to have so many wonderful and supportive family members and friends in our life, and it is hard to thank you all. Thank you to the ones who said goodbye to us before we left for Perth and prayed we would one day come back with a family of our own. Thank you to those who have been there, supporting us through our fertility struggles and celebrating our joy when Bane and Daya came into our lives. I love seeing the continued joy and laughs so many of you get from having Bane and Daya as a big part of your lives as well. I hope you all get enjoyment

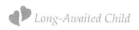

from reading my story.

Lastly, to Bane and Daya: I love you both with all my heart. Bane: your smile, laugh and unconditional love constantly melts my heart. You are such a well-behaved boy and I am so proud of how far you have come. Daya: if you could you would be glued to my side, which at times can drive me a little crazy, but deep down I know you love me more than anything in this world. I get so much enjoyment when we dance around the house together. We have a lot of fun. You both bring so much joy to our lives every day and even though I thought it would not be possible, I love each year with you more than the one before. One day I will sit with you both and share this book with you and explain how beautiful and generous your birth mother, Manu, is. I hope you are proud of your Daddy and I for the journey we had to take to have you and deep down believe we would not have it any other way.

Kellie xx

AUTHOR'S BIOGRAPHY

Kellie grew up in Hervey Bay, Queensland, Australia with her mum, stepdad, sister, and step-sisters. When she was 22 years old, she moved to Port Douglas where she worked in a large resort; it was the start of her career in hotel management. She has had some amazing career opportunities to also work on the Gold Coast, Brisbane, Fraser Island, Perth and the Sunshine Coast, and all the way over to Dublin, Ireland.

Kellie was just shy of 30 when she met Ian. They both worked at the same resort in Noosa Heads on

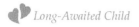

Queensland's Sunshine Coast. After Kellie's eight-year struggle with infertility, she felt compelled to write about her story in the hopes of inspiring other women in similar situations.

Kellie currently lives on the Sunshine Coast with her partner, Ian, and their two children, Bane and Daya. They enjoy spending time at the beach along with socialising with friends and their children.

CONNECT WITH KELLIE

Kellie would love to hear from you about her book and about your journey as well.

To connect with Kellie, go to her website: www.longa-waitedchild.com

Say hi and connect with Kellie on her social media pages:

Facebook: Long Awaited Child

Instagram: Long Awaited Child

BIBLIOGRAPHY

Website links:

Adoption services through the Queensland
Government
https://www.qld.gov.au/community/caring-child/
adopting-child-queensland

Life Fertility (for IVF)
www.lifefertility.com.au

Natural Killer (NK) Cell Testing
IVF Australia
https://www.ivf.com.au/fertility-treatment/
advanced-science/natural-killer-cell-testing

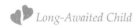

Queensland Fertility Group
https://www.qfg.com.au/fertility-treatment/natu-
ral-killer-cell-testing

Index

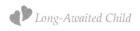

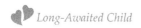

Queensland's Adoption Services 36, 37, 39, 40

S

same sex 45, 79, 133
selective reduction 76
sperm sample 66
surrogacy clinic 57, 64, 65, 74, 77, 82, 88, 130
surrogacy laws 46, 47, 54, 55, 58, 78
surrogate 45, 46, 53, 54, 55, 58, 64, 66, 67, 68, 69, 70, 71, 76,
        78, 79, 82, 104, 110, 116, 127, 130, 133, 134, 142

T

twins 33, 75, 77, 79, 80, 84, 93, 97, 103, 106, 116, 121, 122,
        124, 126, 130, 135, 142, 145

U

uterine cysts 48

V

Vitamin D 120

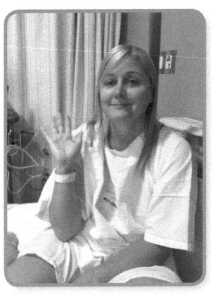

Kellie going in for IVF egg retrieval surgery in Perth.

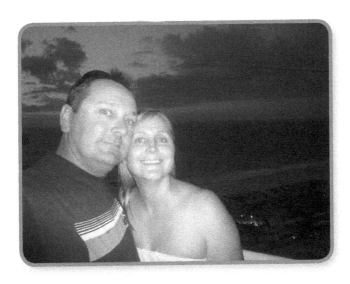

Ian and Kellie enjoying News Years Eve at the hotel Kellie worked at in Perth—knowing we were going to be parents in a few months time.

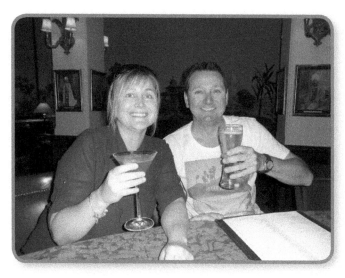

Kellie and Ian enjoying a much needed drink at the Imperial Hotel bar in New Delhi after their first visit to the clinic.

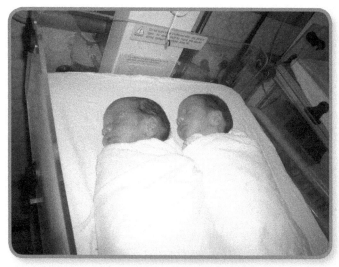

Bane and Daya in their crib at the hospital, and the first Kellie and Ian saw them.

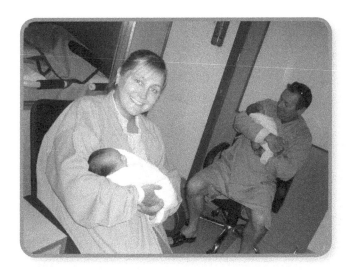

Kellie holding Bane and Ian holding Daya—the first time they held them.

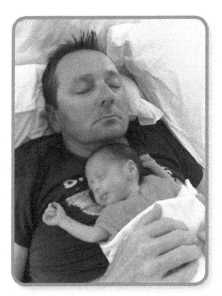

Ian asleep with tiny Daya on the bed in the hotel in New Delhi.

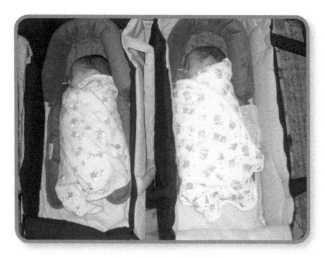

Bane and Daya in their Phil & Ted's cocoons Ian and Kellie carried them in around New Delhi.

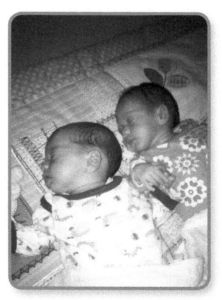

Back in Perth—photo of Bane & Daya that Kellie posted on Facebook introducing them to family and friends.

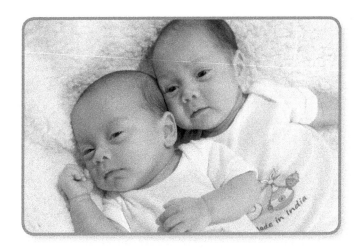

Professional photo of Bane and Daya in their "made in India" jumpsuits.

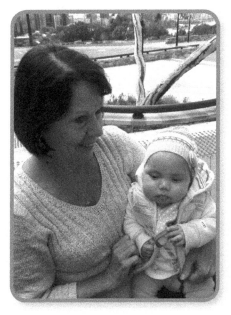

Daya with her Granny when she visited us in Perth.

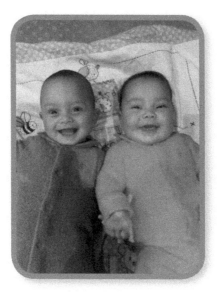

A photo Kellie loves of Bane and Daya at a few months old and loving life already.

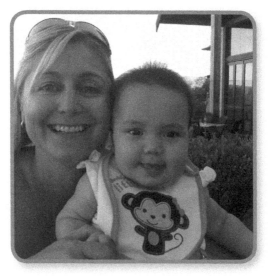

Kellie and Daya on Kellie's 40th birthday.

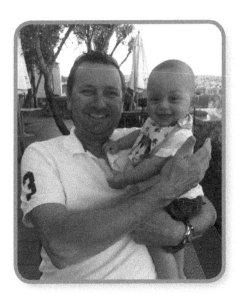

Ian and Bane on Kellie's 40th birthday.

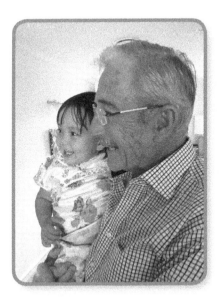

Living back in Queensland. Daya and her Pa (Daya 18months).

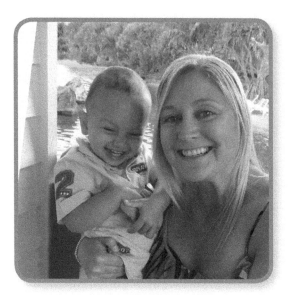

Bane & Kellie (Bane 18months).

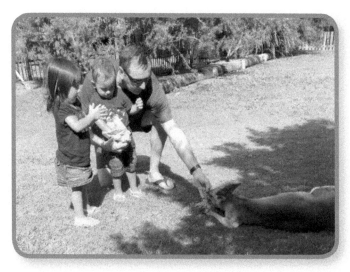

Ian & Bane feeding Kangaroo.

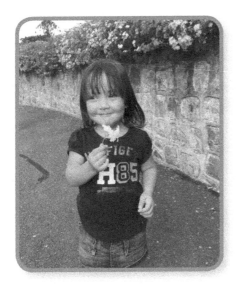

Daya aged 2.

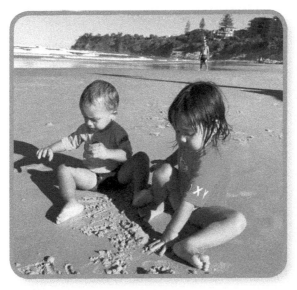

Loving beach life (aged 2)

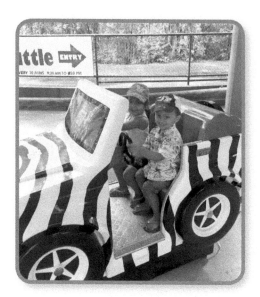

3rd birthday at Australia Zoo

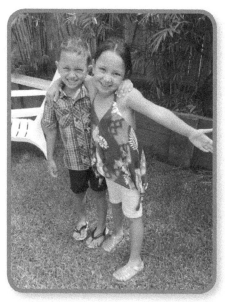

Bane and Daya best friends aged 4.

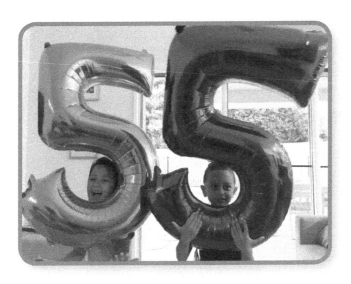

Bane and Daya's 5th birthday

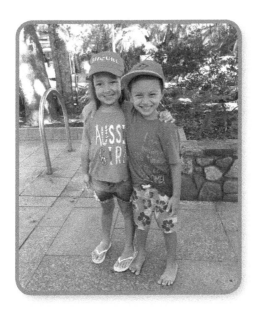

Bane and Daya enjoying life on the Sunshine Coast aged 5

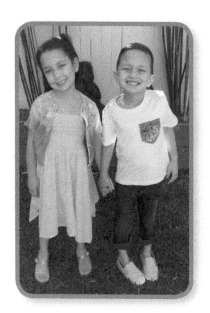

Daya and Bane aged 5

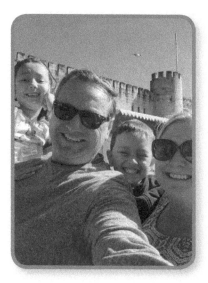

Family day out on the Sunshine Coast